Cooking
with the
Diabetic
Chef

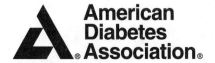

American
Diabetes
Association®

CHRIS SMITH

Text Design and Composition, Circle Graphics; Cover Design, Wickham & Associates, Inc.; Nutrient Analysis, Nutritional Solutions; Printer, Port City Press, Inc.

Printed in the United States of America
3 5 7 9 10 8 6 4

The suggestions and information contained in this publication are generally consistent with the Clinical Practice Recommendations and other policies of the American Diabetes Association, but they do not represent the policy or position of the Association or any of its boards or committees. Reasonable steps have been taken to ensure the accuracy of the information presented. However, the American Diabetes Association cannot ensure the safety or efficacy of any product or service described in this publication. Individuals are advised to consult a physician or other appropriate health care professional before undertaking any diet or exercise program or taking any medication referred to in this publication. Professionals must use and apply their own professional judgment, experience, and training and should not rely solely on the information contained in this publication before prescribing any diet, exercise, or medication. The American Diabetes Association—its officers, directors, employees, volunteers, and members—assumes no responsibility or liability for personal or other injury, loss, or damage that may result from the suggestions or information in this publication.

♾ The paper in this publication meets the requirements of the ANSI Standard Z39.48-1992 (permanence of paper).

ADA titles may be purchased for business or promotional use or for special sales. To purchase this book in large quantities, or for custom editions of this book with your logo, contact Lee Romano Sequeira, Special Sales & Promotions, at the address below, or at LRomano@diabetes.org or 703-299-2046.

American Diabetes Association
1701 North Beauregard Street
Alexandria, VA 22311

Library of Congress Cataloging-in-Publication Data

Smith, Christopher J., 1966–
    Cooking with the diabetic chef / Christopher J. Smith.
      p. cm.
    Includes index.
    ISBN 1-58040-043-4 (pbk. : alk. paper)
    1. Diabetes—Diet therapy—Recipes.   I. Title.

RC662 .S577 2000
641.5'6314—dc21
                                                      00-036208

For my parents.
Thank you for your love and constant support. This book is
dedicated to you both.

Thanks also to the staff of the American Diabetes Association, especially:
Robert J. Anthony, for your guidance and direction, Peter Banks, Len Boswell,
Lee Romano Sequeira, and Marcia Mazur.

Contents

Summer

*F*all

*W*inter

Foreword

I love food! I remember the first seminar I ever gave as if it was yesterday. I was living in New York at the time, where my endocrinologists were Dr. Katsiff and Dr. Gray. I had been under their care for a number of months when Dr. Gray asked if I would be interested in speaking to the local diabetes support group at New York University. With my background, Dr. Gray thought I could provide tips on cooking for people with diabetes.

I agreed to speak and started to create some basic lessons that would allow people to understand the classic techniques for creating great-tasting food. As I worked on these lessons, I became more excited. This seminar would let me share not only my love of food but also my knowledge of cooking with people who genuinely needed a different approach to meal planning.

As the day of the seminar approached, I felt a new sense of calm. I realized that I was at ease because I had thoroughly prepared for this event. I kept reviewing in my own head the topics I would discuss, the questions I thought people would ask—I even pictured myself saying goodnight to the audience after a successful talk. I was sure that I had thought of everything.

When I entered the room, I began to set up my displays and the assortment of things that I had brought with me on healthy eating habits. People started to arrive. Most of them were older people with type 2 diabetes. Before I knew what was happening the room was overflowing, and the organizers were searching around for more chairs. Pretty soon it was standing room only. There were even people lined up in the doorway. I began to speak to the crowd.

There is no greater compliment to a chef than to be in the presence of people who want to know more about food and cooking. I felt that I had entered a world that was very exciting and full of interaction. I spoke about nutrition and different cooking techniques. The audience responded with interest, asking about different flavors and the things they could or could not eat. I felt very confident because I had expected all of these questions and could answer them easily.

Then an unexpected question came. A man in the audience stood up and began to criticize. "You're a chef," he said. "Maybe *you* can make these dishes, but the everyday person can't do this!"

I tried to assure the man that the everyday person could, but he resisted, saying, "I don't have the time to do what you're talking about!"

I thought I had prepared for everything, but I had never counted on this. My mind searched quickly for an answer. Finally I asked him a direct question. Why had he attended this seminar in the first place?

"I want to eat good food," he explained simply.

At this point I turned to address the entire audience. "We all have a disease called diabetes. With this disease, after blood glucose control, food management is the most important factor in our continued health. We all can enjoy food. But to do this we all need the tools to succeed. It all starts with an understanding of food—the techniques of cooking, different ingredients, flavors, portion control, and a balanced meal plan. Once we have these tools, then we can create flavorful food."

When I explained myself this way, the man who had been objecting understood what I was trying to do.

As I left that night, I felt an overwhelming feeling of satisfaction at being able to share my thoughts with this group of people. On the drive home, I thought about what people with diabetes need and how a chef could really meet those needs. I quickly realized that this was what I really wanted to do with my life. From that moment on, I started to prepare for my role as *The Diabetic Chef*.

$\mathcal{I}$ntroduction

My Story

Everything in my life was going according to plan. I was midway through the famed Culinary Institute of America and apprenticing at one of New York's most prestigious restaurants, Le Cirque. But my path to being a great chef was about to take a different turn.

Le Cirque was no different than any four-star restaurant. The schedule was demanding. All the chefs worked six days each week and well over eight hours each day. Although the Culinary Institute of America had an excellent curriculum, nothing could have prepared me for working in a restaurant except actual experience. I was surrounded by some of the best chefs in the country. Whenever they asked me to do something, I did not hesitate. I prepared vegetables, assisted the cooks, whatever it took. To me this was a learning experience, and I wanted to absorb everything I could.

The restaurant kitchen is a fast-paced environment with everyone constantly moving. Although I was used to such a pace, I soon felt fatigued and run down. It was strange. I had always been energetic and had never tired easily. The first week I tried to ignore it. I assumed it was because of the newness of the work and the long commute I took each day to get to the restaurant.

By the third week, however, I could no longer continue. Not only was I completely drained, but I noticed that I was constantly thirsty and needed to urinate more and more frequently. I just could not keep up with the job, and the work was beginning to suffer. I approached the head chef of the restaurant and resigned that very night. I decided to take my experience at Le Cirque for a learning experience and to finish my apprenticeship at a restaurant closer to home.

When I returned to the Culinary Institute of America for my fourth semester, the feeling of fatigue only deepened. Besides the frequent thirst and urination, I started to develop stomach pains and cramps. I finally went to a doctor to find out what was wrong with me. At first no one was sure what it was. The doctor treated me for an ulcer, but my symptoms still persisted. Months later, after my weight had dropped by about 30 pounds, the doctor suggested a test for diabetes. With a simple prick of the finger, the initial diagnosis was made. I returned the following day for a fasting glucose test, and the diagnosis was confirmed. I had type 1 diabetes.

Since my mother was the Director of Surgical Nursing at a hospital on Long Island, I went to see her. She introduced me to some of the medical staff. They told me the greatest news I could have wanted to hear, that I could keep my diabetes in control. With proper care and insulin management, my life would not have to change radically. With the help of a diabetes educator and a registered dietitian, I armed myself with the knowledge I would need for the future. It was such a relief to me to know that I could continue to pursue my dreams.

I returned to the Culinary Institute of America for my final semester. Though I was worried about what the future with diabetes might bring, I took a chance as a chef in the Garden City Hotel, the only four-star hotel on Long Island. There I began to learn in earnest about food, the importance not only of taste but of presentation. And I also learned about managing my diabetes even under the most hectic conditions. If I could do that, I knew I could do anything.

Healthy Eating with Diabetes

If I asked how many people enjoy food, I am sure the response would be pretty high. But if I asked how many people enjoy healthy food, I doubt the numbers would be as promising. To most people "healthy" food means "flavorless" food. But that does not have to be the case.

My approach to food is simple: Get back to the basics. Ingredients should be as natural and fresh as possible. Select meat and seafood that has not been previously frozen. Buy the most fresh and ripe fruits and vegetables.

Then use traditional cooking techniques to bring out the best flavors of those ingredients. A number of classic techniques have been included in these recipes. Though they have been adapted for the ease of the home cook, these techniques have stood the test of time and are the best of the best. They might seem complex at first, but you will see that there really isn't anything here that you can't, or haven't already, done. So give it a try and have fun!

A Note about Food Labels

Many food labels in the grocery store use terms that can be confusing. To help you shop and eat better, here is a list of the common terms as defined by the Food and Drug Administration.

Sugar

Sugar Free: Less than 0.5 gram of sugar per serving.
No Added Sugar, Without Added Sugar, No Sugar Added: This does not mean the same as "sugar free." A label bearing these words means that no sugars were added during processing, or that processing does not increase the sugar content above the amount the ingredients naturally contain. Consult the nutrition information panel to see the total amount of sugar in this product.
Reduced Sugar: At least 25% less sugar per serving than the regular product.

Calories

Calorie Free: Fewer than 5 calories per serving.
Low Calorie: 40 calories or less per serving. (If servings are smaller than 30 grams, or smaller than 2 tablespoons, this means 40 calories or less per 50 grams of food.)
Reduced Calorie, Fewer Calories: At least 25% fewer calories per serving than the regular product.

Fat

Fat Free, Nonfat: Less than 0.5 gram of fat per serving.
Low Fat: 3 grams or less of fat per serving. (If servings are smaller than 30 grams, or smaller than 2 tablespoons, this means 3 grams or less of fat per 50 grams of food.)
Reduced Fat, Less Fat: At least 25% less fat per serving than the regular product.

Cholesterol

Cholesterol Free: Less than 2 milligrams of cholesterol, and 2 grams or less of saturated fat per serving.

Low Cholesterol: 20 milligrams or less of cholesterol, and 2 grams or less of saturated fat per serving.

Reduced Cholesterol, Less Cholesterol: At least 25% less cholesterol, and 2 grams or less of saturated fat per serving than the regular product.

Sodium

Sodium Free: Less than 5 milligrams of sodium per serving.

Low Sodium: 140 milligrams or less of sodium per serving.

Very Low Sodium: 35 milligrams or less of sodium per serving.

Reduced Sodium, Less Sodium: At least 25% less sodium per serving than the regular product.

Light or Lite Foods

Foods that are labeled "Light" or "Lite" are usually either lower in fat or lower in calories than the regular product. Some products may also be lower in sodium. Check the nutrition information label on the back of the product to make sure.

Meat and Poultry

Lean: Less than 10 grams of fat, 4.5 grams or less of saturated fat, and less than 95 milligrams of cholesterol per serving and per 100 grams.

Extra Lean: Less than 5 grams of fat, less than 2 grams of saturated fat, and less than 95 milligrams of cholesterol per serving and per 100 grams.

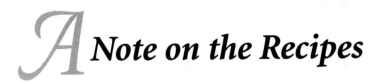 Note on the Recipes

Herbs and Spices

Throughout the book you will see lots of herbs and spices used. Sometimes a recipe will ask for "fresh rosemary," for example. Other times the recipe may only ask for "rosemary." Unless otherwise indicated, use dried spices in the recipes.

Fat Content

Some of the recipes contain higher amounts of fat than usual. Does this mean you should avoid them? Not necessarily. Try to practice balance in your meal planning. For example, if you know you will be having a dinner that is higher in fat, try to make your breakfast and lunch very low in fat. This will help you keep your daily fat intake to an acceptable level.

For those people with high cholesterol levels or at significant risk for heart disease, a reduction of fat intake is even more important. Talk with your doctor to determine a diet that will work for you. You could even bring this book along and ask your doctor which recipes would be best for you.

Spring

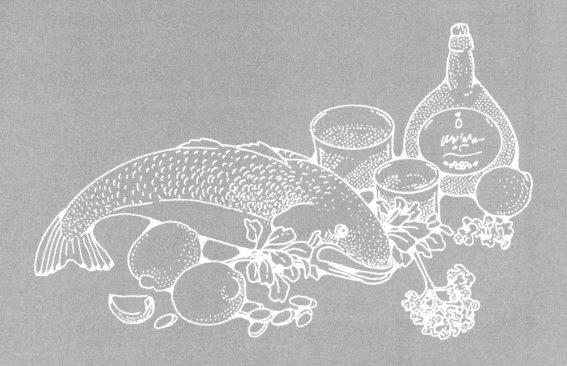

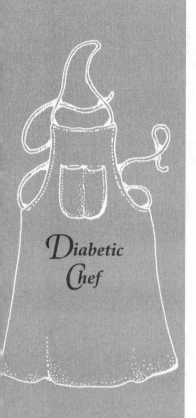

Diabetic Chef

Great food starts with great ingredients. Using the freshest meats and vegetables will make a big difference in the final dish. With spring in the air, it's a wonderful time to take advantage of all the fresh produce that becomes available.

Across the country, chefs will be visiting the local farmers for the freshest ingredients. Chefs know to steer clear of the larger produce companies when they can find great taste and quality in their own communities. You can probably do the same. Many areas have farmers markets where local growers can display and sell their produce.

With freshness in mind, I have created recipes that are light but full of flavor. From the *Sautéed Lemon Shrimp with Zucchini and Yellow Squash Julienne* to the *Lima Bean, Corn, and Green Bean Toss*, I use only those ingredients that are at their peak of freshness. With a simple *Sautéed Spinach* you can enjoy the true flavor of the produce. Or with the *Raspberry Peach Tartlets* you can taste the marriage of truly different and delicious flavors.

Texas French Toast

Ingredients

3 large eggs
6 Tbsp low-fat (1%) milk
1 vanilla bean, pulp
   removed
1 tsp ground cinnamon
   Nonstick cooking spray
4 slices white bread,
   thick-cut

4 Servings
Serving Size: 1 slice

Calories	150
Calories from Fat	48
Total Fat	5 g
Saturated Fat	2 g
Cholesterol	161 mg
Sodium	220 mg
Carbohydrate	17 g
Dietary Fiber	1 g
Sugars	3 g
Protein	8 g

Exchanges

1 Starch
1 Lean Meat
1/2 Fat

Preparation

1. In a large bowl, whisk together the eggs, milk, vanilla bean, and cinnamon.
2. Spray a nonstick pan with cooking spray, and heat it over the stove on medium.
3. Dip the bread slices into the egg batter and place them in the pan. Cook one side until golden brown, then turn the slices over and cook the remaining side until golden brown. Serve with the Vanilla Butter recipe on p. 154.

*S*outhwestern Grits

Ingredients

- 2 cups water
- 4 oz instant grits
- 1/2 Tbsp jalapeño peppers, minced and seeded
- 1/2 Tbsp ground cumin
- 1/4 cup red onion, diced
- 1/4 cup red bell pepper, seeded and diced
- 3 oz sharp cheddar, shredded

4 Servings
Serving Size: 6 oz

Calories	194
Calories from Fat	68
Total Fat	7.5 g
Saturated Fat	4.5 g
Cholesterol	22 mg
Sodium	445 mg
Carbohydrate	25 g
Dietary Fiber	2 g
Sugars	1.5 g
Protein	8 g

Exchanges
1 Starch
1 Lean Meat
1 Fat

Preparation

1. Place water in a heavy saucepan and bring to a boil. Slowly add the grits to water while stirring, bring to a simmer, then lower heat to medium. Add the jalapeños, cumin, red onion, and red pepper, and combine well. The grits should be cooked almost immediately. Remove from heat, garnish with the cheddar cheese, and serve.

Beef Stir-fry

Ingredients

1 Tbsp sesame oil
1 lb sirloin or top round beef, thinly sliced
1 medium red bell pepper, julienned
1 medium yellow bell pepper, julienned
1 medium carrot, julienned
1 Tbsp garlic, minced
1 Tbsp fresh ginger, grated
1 red onion, thinly sliced
1 cup broccoli florets
2 Tbsp cornstarch
2 Tbsp water
2 Tbsp rice wine vinegar
3 Tbsp soy sauce
3 cups cooked white rice
4 green onions, chopped
1 Tbsp sesame seeds, toasted

6 Servings

Serving Size: 1/2 cup stir-fry over 1/2 cup rice

Calories	343
Calories from Fat	79
Total Fat	9 g
Saturated Fat	3 g
Cholesterol	67 mg
Sodium	520 mg
Carbohydrate	36 g
Dietary Fiber	2 g
Sugars	3.5 g
Protein	28 g

Exchanges

2 Starch
3 Very Lean Meat
1 Vegetable
1 Fat

Preparation

1. Place the pan (or wok) on high heat. Add 3/4 of the sesame oil and half of the beef and stir continuously. Cook for about 4–5 minutes, or until the beef is thoroughly done. Remove the beef from the pan, add the rest of your meat, and repeat. Set the cooked beef aside on a separate plate.
2. Add the rest of the sesame oil. Add red and yellow bell peppers. Stir continuously for about 1 minute. Add the carrots, garlic, ginger, red onions, and broccoli florets. Continue to stir until the vegetables are tender, about 3–5 minutes.
3. In a small bowl, whisk together the cornstarch and water until it forms a smooth paste. Add the rice wine vinegar and the soy sauce to the pan. Slowly pour the cornstarch mixture into the pan and toss the ingredients to combine and thicken the sauce. Add the cooked beef to the pan. Continue to toss all the ingredients until they are coated with the sauce.
4. Serve over 1/2 cup of cooked white rice and garnish with green onions and toasted sesame seeds.

Chef's Hints: For a good stir fry, the secret is high heat. Everything should be prepared ahead of time and ready for use. Make sure you cut all of your ingredients thin so that they will cook quickly. Always keep the food in your pan (or a wok, if you have one) moving by stirring.

Flavor Idea: Toasted sesame seeds can add an extra dimension of flavor to a stir-fry, and it is easy to do. Either place the sesame seeds underneath a broiler for a few minutes, or put them in a pan over medium heat. Cook them until they are just lightly browned.

Asparagus Wrapped in Phyllo

Ingredients

- 2 quarts water
- 1/2 lb asparagus
- 1 tsp salt
- 3 sheets store-bought phyllo dough
- 3 Tbsp butter, melted
- 4 tsp Parmesan cheese, grated

---

4 Servings
Serving Size: 1 triangle

Calories	115
Calories from Fat	49
Total Fat	7 g
Saturated Fat	4 g
Cholesterol	17 mg
Sodium	114 mg
Carbohydrate	10 g
Dietary Fiber	1 g
Sugars	1 g
Protein	3 g

Exchanges
1/2 Starch
1/2 Vegetable
1 Fat

Preparation

1. Preheat the oven to 350°F. Bring the water to a boil in a large pot. Trim 1 inch off the bottoms of the asparagus stalks. Add the asparagus heads and the salt to the boiling water. Cook for 1–3 minutes, or until the asparagus is tender. Drain and run the asparagus under cold water. Pat dry.
2. Lay one layer of the phyllo dough on the counter and brush one side with the melted butter. Place the second layer of dough directly overtop and brush with butter again. Repeat for the third layer. Cut the phyllo evenly in quarters.
3. Place 4–6 stalks of asparagus on one of the pieces of layered phyllo. Sprinkle 1 tsp of the Parmesan cheese overtop, then fold the phyllo dough over the asparagus so that it forms a triangle. Seal the edges gently with fingertips. Lightly coat the tops of the triangles with butter.
4. Bake the phyllo in the oven for about 20 minutes, or until the phyllo dough is golden brown. Serve immediately.

Chef's Hints: Choose asparagus stalks that are green with the tips tightly closed. Avoid any stalks with white spots or stalks that are flat. Never purchase fresh asparagus if it is being stored in water. The ideal time to purchase asparagus is between March and June.

Chicken and Mushrooms in White Wine Sauce

Ingredients

4 boneless, skinless chicken breasts
1 tsp salt
1 tsp black pepper
2 tsp garlic powder
2 tsp ground sage
1 cup all-purpose flour
  Nonstick cooking spray
1 cup Shitake mushrooms, sliced
2 cups white mushrooms, sliced
2 Tbsp shallots, finely chopped
2 cups white wine
2 cups Chicken Stock (see p. 155)
3 Tbsp cornstarch
3 Tbsp cold water
2 Tbsp parsley, chopped

4 Servings

Serving Size: 1 chicken breast with 1/4 cup sauce

Calories	157
Calories from Fat	28
Total Fat	3 g
Saturated Fat	1 g
Cholesterol	73 mg
Sodium	135 mg
Carbohydrate	2 g
Dietary Fiber	0 g
Sugars	0 g
Protein	27 g

Exchanges

3 Very Lean Meat
1/2 Fat

Preparation

1. Preheat the oven to 350°F. Season the chicken with the salt, black pepper, garlic powder, and ground sage. Put the flour in a separate, shallow bowl, then dredge the chicken breasts through the flour until they are coated. Spray a pan with non-stick cooking spray and place it over medium heat. Place the chicken breasts in the pan, allow them to brown on one side. Turn the chicken, then brown the remaining side.

2. Remove the chicken breasts to a baking sheet, and place the sheet in the oven. Cook for 20 minutes (internal temperature of 160°F).

3. While the chicken is cooking, prepare the sauce. Spray the pan used to cook the chicken breasts with nonstick cooking spray, add the mushrooms, and cook over medium heat until the mushrooms are slightly wilted. Add the shallots and cook, stirring continuously, until the shallots are translucent. Add the white wine and allow it to simmer until the pan is nearly dry again. Add the chicken stock and return the liquid to a simmer.

4. In a separate bowl, mix together the cornstarch and the water until it forms a smooth paste. Slowly pour the corn-starch mixture into the simmering liquid, and whisk until the sauce thickens. Return the liquid to a simmer, then remove it from the heat. Pour sauce over chicken, sprinkle with parsley, and serve.

Chef's Hints: Using white wine in a sauce gives added taste. The alcohol in the wine evaporates during the cooking, and so do the calories. Sometimes, though, the alcohol can catch fire from the heat. If that happens, do not panic. Simply cover the pan with a lid for a minute to put the flames out.

Chicken Breast Roulade Stuffed with Ham and Goat Cheese

Ingredients

- 4 boneless, skinless chicken breasts
- 1 tsp salt
- 1 tsp white pepper
- 2 slices low-fat ham
- 4 oz goat cheese
- 1/2 cup all-purpose flour
- 1 Tbsp olive oil
- 6 Tbsp Chicken Stock (see p. 155)
- 1 sprig fresh rosemary, chopped
- 2 sprigs fresh thyme, chopped
- 1 sprig fresh oregano, chopped
- 6 fresh chives, chopped

4 Servings

Serving Size: 1 chicken breast with 1 1/2 Tbsp broth

Calories	353
Calories from Fat	178
Total Fat	18 g
Saturated Fat	8 g
Cholesterol	109 mg
Sodium	1197 mg
Carbohydrate	3.5 g
Dietary Fiber	0 g
Sugars	1 g
Protein	39 g

Exchanges

4 Very Lean Meat
1 Lean Meat
3 Fat

Preparation

1. Preheat the oven to 350°F. Using a mallet or meat tenderizer, pound the chicken breasts until they are very thin. Season both sides with salt and white pepper. Place 1 slice of the ham and 1 oz of the goat cheese in the center of each breast. Roll each chicken breast from the end, and secure with a toothpick. Be sure there are no openings where the ingredients can leak out.
2. Put the flour in a separate, shallow bowl, then dredge the chicken breasts through the flour until they are coated. Heat the olive oil in a pan over medium heat. Add the chicken breasts and brown on one side. Flip the chicken breasts to brown the remaining side.
3. Remove the chicken breasts to a baking sheet, and place the sheet in the oven. Cook for 15 minutes (internal temperature of 160°F).
4. While the chicken is cooking, bring the chicken stock to a simmer in a separate pan. Allow it to reduce by half. Just before serving, add the herbs to the stock. Serve the chicken breasts with the herb broth.

Chicken Jambo

Ingredients

- 1/2 Tbsp olive oil
- 2 oz pork sausage, diced
- 1 boneless, skinless chicken breast, chopped
- 1/4 lb large shrimp, deveined, without shells
- 1/2 medium onion, diced
- 1/2 Tbsp garlic, finely chopped
- 1/2 red bell pepper, diced
- 1/2 green bell pepper, diced
- 1/2 cup white wine
- 1 cup long grain white rice
- 2 cups Chicken Stock (see p. 155)
- 1/4 cup fresh tomato, diced
- 1/2 tsp fresh thyme, chopped
- 1/2 tsp fresh oregano, chopped
- 1/2 Tbsp fresh parsley, chopped

5 Servings
Serving Size: 2/3 cup

Calories	257
Calories from Fat	52
Total Fat	6 g
Saturated Fat	1.5 g
Cholesterol	52 mg
Sodium	134 mg
Carbohydrate	34 g
Dietary Fiber	1 g
Sugars	2 g
Protein	13 g

Exchanges

2 Starch
1 Very Lean Meat
1 Vegetable
1 Fat

Preparation

1. Heat olive oil in a pan over medium-high heat. Add sausage and cook 3–4 minutes. Add chicken. Continue to cook until the sausage and chicken are fully cooked, about 8–10 minutes. Remove the chicken and sausage from the pan. Add the shrimp and cook until it is opaque, about 3–4 minutes. Remove the shrimp from the pan.
2. Add the onion, garlic, and red and green peppers and cook for about 3–4 minutes. Add the white wine, and allow the liquid to simmer until it is reduced by half. Add the rice, chicken stock, and tomato, and bring the liquid to a boil. Immediately when it boils, reduce the heat to a simmer and allow the mixture to cook until the rice is tender, about 20–25 minutes.
3. When the rice is finished, add the cooked chicken, sausage, and shrimp. Add the thyme, oregano, and parsley. Gently stir to incorporate all the ingredients and serve.

*R*oast Leg of Lamb

Ingredients

3 lb boneless leg of lamb, trimmed and tied
1 tsp salt
2 tsp black pepper
1 orange rind, grated
1 Tbsp garlic, minced
2 sprigs fresh rosemary
1 Tbsp olive oil

10 Servings
Serving Size: 1 5-oz slice

Calories	266
Calories from Fat	104
Total Fat	12 g
Saturated Fat	4 g
Cholesterol	116 mg
Sodium	322 mg
Carbohydrate	1 g
Dietary Fiber	0 g
Sugars	0 g
Protein	37 g

Exchanges
5 Very Lean Meat
2 Fat

Preparation

1. Season the lamb with the salt, black pepper, grated orange rind, and minced garlic. Place the two rosemary sprigs beneath the butcher's twine so that they rest against the meat. Rub the olive oil over the lamb.
2. Preheat the oven to 350°F. Preheat a large, nonstick pan to medium heat. Spray with a nonstick oil and sear lamb on all sides until golden brown. Place a large pan over medium heat, and place the lamb into it. Cook the lamb on all sides until it is a golden brown. Place the lamb into a roasting pan or dish and put it into the oven. Cook for 1 1/2–2 hours, or to an internal temperature of 160°F. When the lamb is done, allow it to rest for 5–10 minutes out of the oven before serving.

Chef's Hints: Tying a leg of lamb is not always the easiest thing to do for most people. Luckily, many grocery stores sell the boneless leg of lamb already tied. If you cannot find one, ask the butcher at your local grocery store to do it for you.

$\mathcal{V}$eal Scallopini

Ingredients

4	4-oz veal cutlets
1/2	cup all-purpose flour
1	tsp salt
1	tsp black pepper
2	Tbsp olive oil
1	cup white wine
1 1/2	cups canned plum tomatoes, chopped
1	Tbsp capers
1	Tbsp fresh parsley, chopped

4 Servings
Serving Size: 1 veal cutlet with 1/2 cup sauce

Calories	284
Calories from Fat	99
Total Fat	11 g
Saturated Fat	2 g
Cholesterol	95 mg
Sodium	865 mg
Carbohydrate	7 g
Dietary Fiber	1 g
Sugars	2 g
Protein	31 g

Exchanges
4 1/2 Very Lean Meat
2 Fat
1 Vegetable

Preparation

1. If the veal cutlets are not already pounded thin, use a mallet or meat tenderizer to do it yourself. Place the flour, salt, and pepper in a separate, shallow bowl, then dredge the veal cutlets until they are thoroughly coated.
2. Heat the olive oil in a pan over medium heat. Add the veal. When one side is browned, turn the veal over and brown the remaining side. Once both sides are browned, remove the veal from the pan and pat dry with paper towels to remove some of the excess fat.
3. Add white wine to the pan and bring it to a simmer. Allow the liquid to reduce by half. Add the chopped tomatoes and return the liquid to a simmer. Add the capers and simmer for 5 minutes. Add the veal and cook just until it is reheated. Serve immediately and garnish with the chopped parsley.

Orzo Pasta with Baby Shrimp, Sun-Dried Tomatoes, and Sweet Pea Puree

Ingredients

1 Tbsp olive oil
1/2 Tbsp garlic, chopped
2 cups Chicken Stock (see p. 155)
1/2 lb frozen peas
2 quarts water
1/2 lb orzo pasta
1 tsp salt
1 Tbsp olive oil
1/2 lb baby shrimp, deveined and without shells
1/2 cup shallots, chopped
1/2 cup sun-dried tomatoes, chopped

5 Servings
Serving Size: 1 cup

Calories	287
Calories from Fat	36
Total Fat	4 g
Saturated Fat	.5 g
Cholesterol	65 mg
Sodium	136 mg
Carbohydrate	47 g
Dietary Fiber	4 g
Sugars	6.5 g
Protein	16 g

Exchanges
2 1/2 Starch
1 Very Lean Meat
1 Vegetable
1/2 Fat

Preparation

1. In a medium pot, heat the olive oil over medium heat. Add the garlic and stir until it turns opaque. Add the chicken stock and peas. Bring to a simmer for 15 minutes, then remove from heat. Place the mixture into a blender or food processor and blend until smooth.
2. In a large pot, bring the 2 quarts of water to a boil. Add the orzo pasta and the salt. Stir immediately to prevent the pasta from sticking. Cook until the pasta is done, about 10–12 minutes.
3. Heat the olive oil in a large pan over medium-high heat. Add shrimp and shallots and stir quickly to cook. When the shrimp has turned opaque, add the sun-dried tomatoes and toss gently.
4. Mix the pasta and pea puree. Serve the pasta with the shrimp mixture on top.

Chef's Hints: Cooking the pasta in advance can save you time while you prepare the rest of the recipe.

Fresh Steamed Clams and Mussels with Spicy Marinara over Orechetta Pasta

Ingredients

1 lb orechetta pasta
1 gallon water
1 Tbsp garlic, chopped
1 Tbsp butter
1 cup water
1 lb fresh clams
1 lb mussels
3 cups Spicy Marinara Sauce (see p. 148)
1 bunch fresh parsley, chopped

5 Servings
Serving Size: 1/2 cup pasta, 1/4 sauce

Calories	336
Calories from Fat	42
Total Fat	5 g
Saturated Fat	1 g
Cholesterol	51 mg
Sodium	422 mg
Carbohydrate	45 g
Dietary Fiber	3 g
Sugars	9 g
Protein	28 g

Exchanges
2 Starch
3 Lean Meat
1 1/2 Vegetable
1/2 Fat

Preparation

1. In a medium pot, bring the water to a boil. Add the orechetta pasta, and stir immediately to prevent the pasta from sticking. Cook until the pasta is done, about 10–12 minutes.
2. In a large pot, bring the water, garlic, and butter to a boil. Thoroughly rinse the clams and mussels under cold, running tap water and discard any opened shells. Place the clams and mussels into the boiling water and cover the pot. Steam the clams and mussels for 6–10 minutes, or until done. The clams and mussels are finished cooking when the shells have opened.
3. Remove clams and mussels from pot and reduce liquid by half. Add 3 cups of the Spicy Marinara Sauce and gently stir until all the shells are coated. Arrange the clams and mussels over the cooked pasta, pour the remaining sauce overtop, and garnish with the chopped parsley.

Salmon Roulade

Ingredients

1 whole salmon, skin removed
2 oz Herb Butter (see p. 158)
1 Tbsp fresh thyme, chopped
1 Tbsp fresh rosemary, chopped
2 Tbsp Fresh chives, chopped

6 Servings

Serving Size: 1 salmon roulade

Calories	256
Calories from Fat	132
Total Fat	14.5 g
Saturated Fat	7 g
Cholesterol	101 mg
Sodium	100 mg
Carbohydrate	1 g
Dietary Fiber	0 g
Sugars	0 g
Protein	29 g

Exchanges

4 1/2 Very Lean Meat
2 1/2 Fat

Preparation

1. Preheat the oven to 350°F. Slice the salmon into 1/2–3/4-inch wide pieces lengthwise, so that you end up with 6 long strips of salmon. Roll the pieces from the end into a tight circle. Push a toothpick through the length of the salmon rolls to keep them from unrolling in the oven.
2. Season the salmon rolls with the herb butter, thyme, rosemary, and chives. Place evenly on a baking sheet, and put into the oven. Cook for 20 minutes, or until the fish is done.

*B*aked Sea Scallops

Ingredients

- 2 lb sea scallops
- 2/3 cup white wine
- 2 Tbsp lemon juice
- Black pepper
- 3 cups cooked white rice

6 Servings

Serving Size: 5 oz scallops, 1/2 cup rice

Calories	305
Calories from Fat	45
Total Fat	5 g
Saturated Fat	1 g
Cholesterol	48 mg
Sodium	623 mg
Carbohydrate	31 g
Dietary Fiber	.5 g
Sugars	0 g
Protein	27 g

Exchanges

1 1/2 Starch
3 Very Lean Meat
1 Fat

Preparation

1. Preheat oven to 350°F. Space scallops evenly in a shallow baking dish. Add the white wine and lemon juice. Cook the scallops in the oven for 8–12 minutes, or until fully cooked. Season with black pepper and serve over rice.

Shrimp Salad with Dill and Cucumber

Ingredients

3   quarts water
1   lemon, sliced into wedges
1   tsp whole black peppercorns
2   bay leaves
1 1/2 lb medium shrimp, deveined and without shells
1/2 cup reduced-fat mayonnaise
1/2 cup onion, minced
2   cups cucumber, pealed, seeded, and diced
2   Tbsp fresh dill, chopped

---

6 Servings
Serving Size: about 1/2 cup

Calories	183
Calories from Fat	72
Total Fat	8 g
Saturated Fat	1 g
Cholesterol	228 mg
Sodium	395 mg
Carbohydrate	4 g
Dietary Fiber	1 g
Sugars	0 g
Protein	24 g

Exchanges
3 1/2 Very Lean Meat
1/2 Vegetable
1 Fat

Preparation

1. Bring the water to a boil in a large pot. Add the lemon wedges, peppercorns, and bay leaves. Add the shrimp and cook for 3 minutes, or until the shrimp is fully done. Drain the water and cover with ice water to cool the shrimp.
2. Once the shrimp is cool, drain the water and coarsely chop the shrimp. Combine the shrimp with remaining ingredients. Refrigerate for 1 hour, then serve.

Smoked Salmon with Goat Cheese on Baguette Rounds

Ingredients

1 French baguette
8 oz goat cheese, plain
 or herbed
1/2 lb smoked salmon
2 oz capers
 Fresh dill sprigs

---

8 Servings
Serving Size: 3 pieces

Calories	214
Calories from Fat	95
Total Fat	10.5 g
Saturated Fat	6 g
Cholesterol	29 mg
Sodium	1035 mg
Carbohydrate	15.5 g
Dietary Fiber	1 g
Sugars	1 g
Protein	14 g

Exchanges
1 Starch
1 1/2 Lean Meat
1 Fat

Preparation

1. Preheat oven to 350°F. Slice the baguette into 3/8-inch thick pieces and place in oven for 8–10 minutes, or until lightly toasted. Remove the rounds from the oven and allow them to cool.
2. Spread goat cheese on top of each round. Place a small piece of smoked salmon on top of the goat cheese. Garnish each piece with capers and a small sprig of dill. Arrange on a plate and serve.

Chef's Hints: A 'baguette' is just a fancy name for a hard, thin French bread. You have probably seen these many times in the grocery store. A typical baguette is about a foot and a half long, hard to the touch, and no more than an inch or two across. When cut into rounds, the slices should be about size of a half-dollar.

Sautéed Lemon Shrimp with Zucchini and Yellow Squash Julienne

Ingredients

- 2 medium zucchini
- 2 medium yellow squash
- 1 Tbsp butter
- 1/4 tsp salt
- 1/4 tsp white pepper
  Nonstick cooking spray
- 1 1/2 lb large shrimp, deveined and without shells
- 1 lemon
- 2 Tbsp fresh parsley, chopped

6 Servings

Serving Size: 1/2 cup shrimp, 1/3 cup vegetables

Calories	120
Calories from Fat	27
Total Fat	3 g
Saturated Fat	1.5 g
Cholesterol	167 mg
Sodium	286 mg
Carbohydrate	5 g
Dietary Fiber	2 g
Sugars	2 g
Protein	18 g

Exchanges

2 1/2 Very Lean Meat
1/2 Vegetable
1/2 Fat

Preparation

1. Trim the ends of both the zucchini and yellow squash. Cut the vegetables into long, narrow strips (called 'julienne'). In a large pan, melt the butter over medium-high heat. Add the vegetables. Toss until tender, about 3–5 minutes. Season with salt and pepper.

2. Spray a pan with nonstick cooking spray and heat it over medium heat. Add the shrimp and cook until done, about 3–4 minutes. Squeeze the juice of the lemon into the pan and toss until all the shrimp are coated. Serve the shrimp on top of the julienned vegetables and garnish with the chopped parsley.

Carrot and Ginger Soup

Ingredients

1/2	Tbsp olive oil
1/2	cup shallots, chopped
4	Tbsp fresh ginger, minced
1 1/2	lb carrots, large dice
1	quart Chicken Stock (see p. 155)
1/2	tsp salt
	White pepper
4	Tbsp heavy cream
	Fresh chives, chopped

4 Servings
Serving Size: about 1/2 cup

Calories	105
Calories from Fat	19
Total Fat	2 g
Saturated Fat	>1 g
Cholesterol	0 mg
Sodium	353 mg
Carbohydrate	21 g
Dietary Fiber	5 g
Sugars	12 g
Protein	2 g

Exchanges
4 Vegetable

Preparation

1. In a large pot, heat the olive oil over medium heat. Add the shallots and ginger. Cook until the shallots become translucent. Add the diced carrots and enough chicken stock to cover them. Bring the liquid to a boil, then reduce the heat to a simmer. Skim off any scum or fat which floats to the surface, cover the pot tightly, and cook for 15–20 minutes, or until the carrots are very soft.
2. Place the carrots and chicken stock into a blender or food processor and puree until smooth. Season with salt and white pepper. Serve immediately and garnish with a dollop of heavy cream and fresh chives.

Did You Know? The tops of certain root vegetables like beets and carrots need to be removed before storing. The tops draw much of the moisture away from the vegetable itself, causing the vegetables to become bitter.

$\mathcal{V}$egetable Soup

Ingredients

- 1/2 Tbsp olive oil
- 1/2 medium onion, finely diced
- 1/4 medium carrot, julienned
- 1/4 stalk of celery, finely diced
- 1 clove garlic, minced
- 4 Tbsp leeks, finely diced
- 3 Tbsp canned tomato, chopped
- 1/2 cup cooked lima beans
- 1/4 cup frozen peas
- 1/2 potato, peeled and diced
- 1/4 tsp fresh thyme, minced
- 1/4 tsp fresh rosemary minced
- 1/4 tsp fresh oregano, minced
- 3 cups Chicken Stock (see p. 155)
- 1/4 tsp salt
- Pinch white pepper
- 5 parsley leaves, chopped

4 Servings
Serving Size: 1/2 cup

Calories	98
Calories from Fat	27
Total Fat	3 g
Saturated Fat	1 g
Cholesterol	3 mg
Sodium	264 mg
Carbohydrate	13 g
Dietary Fiber	3 g
Sugars	3 g
Protein	5 g

Exchanges
1/2 Starch
1/2 Vegetable

Preparation

1. Heat the olive oil in a pot over medium heat. Add the onions, carrots, and celery. Cook until the vegetables are slightly wilted. Add the garlic and leeks and continue to cook, stirring constantly. Add the tomato, lima beans, peas, potatoes, thyme, rosemary, oregano, and chicken stock.
2. Bring the liquid to a simmer and allow it to cook for 25–30 minutes, or until the potatoes are tender. Season with the salt and pepper. Serve with parsley on top for a garnish.

*A*ntipasti Salad

Ingredients

1/2 lb ziti pasta
3 quarts water
1/2 green bell pepper, diced
1/2 Tbsp garlic, crushed
2 oz feta cheese
2 Tbsp extra virgin olive oil
1/4 small red onion, diced
1/2 red bell pepper, diced
Black pepper, as needed
5 Tbsp balsamic vinegar

5 Servings
Serving Size: 6 oz

Calories	257
Calories from Fat	81
Total Fat	9 g
Saturated Fat	2 g
Cholesterol	10 mg
Sodium	132 mg
Carbohydrate	36 g
Dietary Fiber	2 g
Sugars	5 g
Protein	7 g

Exchanges
2 Starch
1/2 Vegetable
1 1/2 Fat

Preparation

1. Bring the water to a boil in a large pot. Add the ziti pasta and stir to prevent the pasta from sticking. Cook for 10–12 minutes, or until the pasta is done. Drain the water, then cover the pasta with cold water to cool.
2. Once the pasta has cooled, drain the water. Add the remaining ingredients to the pasta and mix well. Refrigerate for 1 hour, mix again, and serve.

$\mathcal{B}$asmati Rice with Lemon and Thyme

Ingredients

1 1/2 cup water
1/2 tsp salt
3/4 cup basmati rice
1/2 medium lemon
1 Tbsp fresh thyme, chopped
Pinch white pepper

4 Servings
Serving Size: 1/2 cup

Calories	139
Calories from Fat	4
Total Fat	>1 g
Saturated Fat	>1 g
Cholesterol	0 mg
Sodium	293 mg
Carbohydrate	31 g
Dietary Fiber	0 g
Sugars	0 g
Protein	3 g

Exchanges
2 Starch

Preparation

1. In a medium pot, bring the water to a boil. Add the salt and basmati rice. Grate the rind from the lemon and add it to the rice. Squeeze the juice from the lemon into the rice. Bring the liquid to a boil, then reduce heat to a simmer. Cover the pot tightly and cook for 20–25 minutes, or until the rice is tender. Add the thyme and season with white pepper.

*L*ima Beans, Corn, and Green Bean Toss

Ingredients

  1 quart water
2/3 cup frozen lima beans
2/3 cup fresh green beans
2/3 cup frozen or fresh
      yellow corn
  2 tsp butter
  1 tsp black pepper

4 Servings
Serving Size: 1/2 cup

Calories	111
Calories from Fat	21
Total Fat	2 g
Saturated Fat	1 g
Cholesterol	5 mg
Sodium	16 mg
Carbohydrate	20 g
Dietary Fiber	5 g
Sugars	3 g
Protein	5 g

Exchanges
1 Starch
1 Vegetable

Preparation

1. In a large pot, bring the water to a boil. Add the lima beans and cook for 10 minutes. Add the green beans and cook for 5 minutes. Add the corn and finish cooking for 5 more minutes. Drain the liquid, add the butter and black pepper, and toss to mix. Serve immediately.

Chef's Hints: To check if a bean is fully cooked simply squeeze it between your fingers. The bean should be soft and free of any hard core.

Sautéed Julienne Vegetables

Ingredients

Nonstick cooking
spray
1/2 cup carrots, julienned
1/2 cup red bell peppers,
julienned
1/2 cup yellow bell
peppers, julienned
1/2 cup asparagus, cooked
 1 Tbsp garlic, minced
 2 tsp Tarragon Butter
(see p. 150)

4 Servings
Serving Size: 1/2 cup

Calories	108
Calories from Fat	28
Total Fat	3 g
Saturated Fat	2 g
Cholesterol	8 mg
Sodium	8 mg
Carbohydrate	13 g
Dietary Fiber	2.5 g
Sugars	4 g
Protein	3 g

Exchanges
1 1/2 Vegetable
1/2 Fat

Preparation

1. Spray a pan with nonstick cooking spray and place over medium-high heat. Add the carrots and cook for 3 minutes. Add the red and yellow bell peppers and cook for 3 minutes. Lower the heat to medium, add the asparagus and garlic, and cook for 3 more minutes. Melt the Tarragon Butter over the vegetables, toss them, and serve immediately.

Did You Know? The Framingham Heart Study showed that 800 middle-aged men who ate three servings of vegetables each day reduced their risk of stroke by 22%.

Sautéed Spinach

Ingredients

- 1 lb fresh spinach, stems removed
- 1/2 Tbsp extra virgin olive oil
- 1/2 Tbsp butter
- 1 Tbsp shallots, chopped
- 1/4 cup Chicken Stock (see p. 155)
- 1/2 tsp salt
- 1 tsp black pepper

(see p. 155)

4 Servings
Serving Size: 2/3 cup

Calories	102
Calories from Fat	30
Total Fat	3 g
Saturated Fat	2 g
Cholesterol	4 mg
Sodium	705 mg
Carbohydrate	8 g
Dietary Fiber	5 g
Sugars	0 g
Protein	6 g

Exchanges
2 Vegetable

Preparation

1. Clean the spinach in a bowl or sink filled with cold water. Make sure to agitate the leaves to remove any sand or dirt that might cling to the spinach.
2. Heat the olive oil and butter in a pan over medium heat. Add the shallots and cook for about 30 seconds. Add the chicken stock and the spinach, cover tightly, and steam until the spinach is tender, about 3–5 minutes. Remove the spinach from the liquid, season with salt and pepper, and serve.

Chef's Hints: Place a small amount of salt in a sink full cold water when washing your vegetables to remove small grains of sand.

Tomato and Zucchini

Ingredients

- 1 Tbsp olive oil
- 1 Tbsp garlic, minced
- 1 14.5-oz can of diced tomatoes
- 2 medium zucchini, sliced
- 1 tsp fresh rosemary, minced
- 2 tsp fresh oregano, minced
- 1 tsp fresh thyme, minced
- Black pepper

4 Servings
Serving Size: 2/3 cup

Calories	72
Calories from Fat	33
Total Fat	4 g
Saturated Fat	.5 g
Cholesterol	0 mg
Sodium	171 mg
Carbohydrate	10 g
Dietary Fiber	2 g
Sugars	4.5 g
Protein	2 g

Exchanges
1 Vegetable
1/2 Fat

Preparation

1. Heat the olive oil in a pan over medium heat. Add the garlic and cook for about 30 seconds. Add the entire contents (juice and all) from the can of diced tomatoes. Bring to a simmer.
2. Cut the zucchini into 1/4-inch slices and add to the pan. Add the rosemary, oregano, and thyme, and stir occasionally until the zucchini is cooked, about 8–10 minutes. Season with black pepper and serve.

Yogurt with Peach Puree and Fresh Raspberries

Ingredients

8 oz canned, sliced peaches

8 oz fresh raspberries

16 oz plain, reduced-fat yogurt

1 cup walnuts, roughly chopped

4 fresh mint leaves

4 Servings
Serving Size: 9 oz

Calories	297
Calories from Fat	163
Total Fat	18 g
Saturated Fat	2 g
Cholesterol	7 mg
Sodium	83 mg
Carbohydrate	25 g
Dietary Fiber	6 g
Sugars	17 g
Protein	14 g

Exchanges
1 Very Lean Meat
1 Fruit
3 1/2 Fat

Preparation

1. Drain the peaches and puree them in a blender or food processor until smooth. Wash the raspberries.
2. In a small bowl, place one-eighth of the yogurt at the bottom. Place one-eighth of the peach puree on top. Place one-eighth of the raspberries on the peach layer. Repeat this layer, then top with chopped walnuts. Garnish each glass with a few raspberries and a mint leaf.

Chocolate Cake Celebration

Ingredients

2 cups reduced-fat chocolate cake mix
3 medium whole oranges
1 pint fresh or frozen raspberries
2 tsp Grand Marnier liquor (can substitute 2 tsp orange juice)

8 Servings
Serving Size: 1 slice

Calories	202
Calories from Fat	40
Total Fat	4 g
Saturated Fat	1 g
Cholesterol	53 mg
Sodium	293 mg
Carbohydrate	39 g
Dietary Fiber	5 g
Sugars	22 g
Protein	4 g

Exchanges
1 Other Carbohydrate
1/2 Fat

Preparation

1. Prepare the reduced-fat cake mix according to the package directions. Bake one layer in an 8 × 8-inch square pan. Allow the cake to cool, then cut it into 8 equal pieces.
2. Peel the oranges and separate the segments of the orange. Using a small paring knife, remove the white membrane. Discard the seeds. Set the segments aside.
3. Rinse the fresh raspberries under cool water and allow them to dry on a paper towel. (If using frozen raspberries, thaw them slightly, setting them on paper towels to absorb the liquid.)
4. Using a clean pastry brush, 'paint' 2 tsp of Grand Marnier (or orange juice) over the cake slices, allowing the cake to absorb the liquid.
5. Garnish each cake slice with 4 orange segments and 3 raspberries and serve.

Raspberry Peach Tartlets

Ingredients

- 1   8.25-oz can of peaches, packed in water
- 1/8–1/4 tsp almond flavoring to taste (optional)
- 1/4–1/2 tsp cinnamon to taste (optional)
- 14   phyllo-dough mini-tartlet shells, pre-baked
- 1   pint fresh or frozen raspberries
- 2   oz grated semi-sweet chocolate

---

7 Servings

Serving Size: 2 filled tartlet shells

Calories	113
Calories from Fat	41
Total Fat	5 g
Saturated Fat	1 g
Cholesterol	0 mg
Sodium	22 mg
Carbohydrate	17 g
Dietary Fiber	4 g
Sugars	8 g
Protein	2 g

Exchanges

1 Other Carbohydrate
1 Fat

Preparation

1. Drain the peaches and put them into a blender. Add the almond and cinnamon flavoring if you wish. Blend until smooth.
2. Place the pre-baked mini-tartlet shells on a plate. Pour 1 Tbsp of the pureed peach mixture into each shell. Arrange 2–3 raspberries on top of the pureed peaches. Garnish with the grated chocolate and serve.

Summer

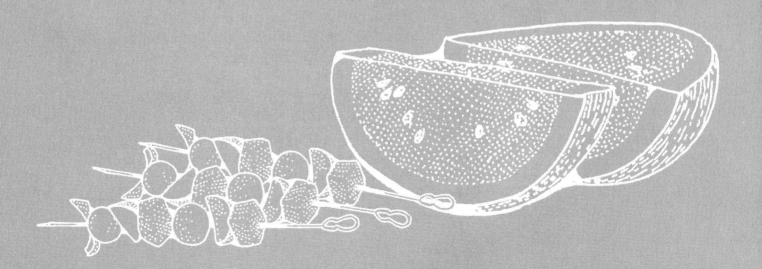

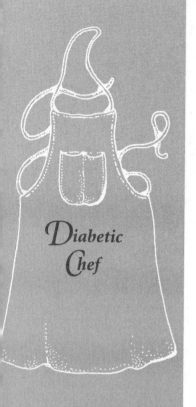

Diabetic Chef

My family would always cook outside during the summer. Just about everything was grilled as we all sat out and enjoyed the warm weather.

Some of my best memories are of my family's July 4th parties. Friends and family would gather to celebrate not only Independence Day but also birthdays and anniversaries. It wasn't uncommon to have 30 or more people in the house, all of them sharing in laughter and conversation.

Everyone would bring a special dish to those parties. Cold salads, barbecued chicken, a watermelon stuffed with fresh fruit. There was always plenty of food to enjoy throughout the day and into the night.

One of my favorite foods was my dad's barbecued ribs. They were delicious. Sweet, but with a hint of spice. The meat was so tender it practically fell off the bone. You can find that recipe right here, *Padre's Country-Style Ribs*. I'm not quite sure where I came up with the nickname, but my dad has always been 'Padre' to me.

Padre was always close to the grill, cooking for all his guests. A line of people would form around him, all of them waiting to be served. The grill became a social area itself, and my dad loved it. As I grew older, I couldn't wait to try my hand at being the 'Grill Man' myself. Now that I'm a chef, I cook on the grill all the time. Try some of the great grill recipes in here—and maybe throw your own July 4th party this year!

Ham and Swiss Mini-quiche

Ingredients

- 3 large eggs
- 1/4 cup ham, diced
- 1/4 cup Swiss cheese, grated
- 2 Tbsp green onions, chopped
- 1/8 tsp black pepper
- 6 frozen mini-quiche shells

4 Servings
Serving Size: about 1 1/2 quiche shells

Calories	294
Calories from Fat	167
Total Fat	19 g
Saturated Fat	3 g
Cholesterol	178 mg
Sodium	582 mg
Carbohydrate	23 g
Dietary Fiber	0 g
Sugars	1 g
Protein	11 g

Exchanges
1 1/2 Other Carbohydrate
1 Lean Meat
3 Fat

Preparation

1. Preheat the oven to 350°F. In a medium-sized bowl, beat together the eggs, ham, Swiss cheese, green onions, and black pepper.
2. Place the quiche shells on a baking sheet, and divide the egg mixture evenly between the quiche shells. Place the quiche shells in the oven and bake for 20–25 minutes, or until firm and lightly browned on top.
3. Remove the quiche shells from the oven and allow them to rest for 2–3 minutes before serving.

Banana and Vanilla Pancakes

Ingredients

2 cups all-purpose flour
1 tsp salt
2 Tbsp sugar
1 tsp baking soda
1 pint reduced-fat (2%)
   milk
2 large eggs, beaten
2 oz butter, melted
1 fresh vanilla bean
1 banana, sliced
   Nonstick cooking spray

6 Servings
Serving Size: 2 pancakes

Calories	322
Calories from Fat	104
Total Fat	12 g
Saturated Fat	6.5 g
Cholesterol	99 mg
Sodium	664 mg
Carbohydrate	45 g
Dietary Fiber	2 g
Sugars	13 g
Protein	9 g

Exchanges
2 Starch
2 Fat

Preparation

1. Sift all the dry ingredients together in a mixing bowl. In a separate bowl, combine the milk, eggs, and butter. Combine the wet and dry ingredients until they form a batter. Slice the vanilla bean in half and scrape out the pulp from the center of the bean. Mix the vanilla pulp into the pancake batter. Gently mix the sliced bananas into the batter.

2. Spray a pan with nonstick cooking spray and heat the pan over medium heat. Use about 1/3 cup of batter per pancake.

Did You Know? If you store an apple near a banana, the banana will ripen in a very short amount of time. This is due to the ethylene gas that apples tend to give off.

_S_ilver-Dollar Sorcery

Ingredients

- 4 Tbsp raisins
- 1/2 cup water, or enough to cover raisins
- 1 cup reduced-calorie pancake mix
- 1 Tbsp reduced-fat semi-sweet chocolate baking chips
- Nonstick cooking spray
- 2 medium apples, peeled and thinly sliced
- 1 vanilla bean (or 1 tsp vanilla extract)
- 1 tsp cinnamon
- 1 Tbsp lite margarine
- 1/4 cup nonfat whipped topping (optional)

4 Servings

Serving Size: 3 pancakes, 1/4 of the sauce

Calories	195
Calories from Fat	31
Total Fat	3 g
Saturated Fat	1 g
Cholesterol	11 mg
Sodium	455 mg
Carbohydrate	41 g
Dietary Fiber	5 g
Sugars	19 g
Protein	6 g

Exchanges

1 1/2 Starch
1 Fruit
1/2 Fat

Preparation

1. Soak the raisins in water (make sure all the raisins are covered) for 30 minutes. (Drain. Reserve the water for later use.) Raisins will plump up.
2. Prepare the pancake mix according to the package directions. Add the semisweet baking chips.
3. Spray a pan with the nonstick spray, then heat the pan over medium-low heat. Sprinkle a few drops of water on the pan. When the water sizzles and disappears, the pan is ready.
4. Drop the pancake mixture onto the hot pan, using a tablespoon to make 12 silver-dollar pancakes. When the pancakes bubble on top, turn and brown them on the other side. When done, remove from the pan.
5. Spray a pan with nonstick spray and place it over low to medium heat. Add the sliced apples and cook 3–5 minutes. Add the raisins, reserved raisin water, vanilla bean (or vanilla extract), and cinnamon. Cook until the liquid is reduced by three-fourths, about 3–5 minutes. Then, stirring the mixture, add the margarine until it is melted.
6. Set 3 warm silver-dollar pancakes on each plate. Spoon the warm apple mixture over the pancakes. Add a dollop of nonfat whipped topping, if you wish. Serve.

Grilled Beef Kabobs

Ingredients

- 1 Tbsp garlic, minced
- 1/2 cup balsamic vinegar
- 2 Tbsp olive oil
- 1 tsp black pepper
- 1 tsp fresh rosemary, minced
- 1 tsp fresh thyme, minced
- 1 lb beef sirloin or top round
- 1 medium red onion, cut into 1/2-inch squares
- 1 large red bell pepper, cut into 1/2-inch squares
- 1 large yellow bell pepper, cut into 1/2-inch squares
- 8 cherry tomatoes

4 Servings
Serving Size: 2 kabobs

Calories	303
Calories from Fat	108
Total Fat	12 g
Saturated Fat	4 g
Cholesterol	101 mg
Sodium	84 mg
Carbohydrate	12 g
Dietary Fiber	2 g
Sugars	6 g
Protein	36 g

Exchanges
4 1/2 Very Lean Meat
2 Vegetable
2 Fat

Preparation

1. Assemble the marinade by combining the garlic, balsamic vinegar, olive oil, black pepper, rosemary, and thyme in a medium bowl.
2. Cut the beef into 1/2–3/4 inch cubes. Place the beef in the marinade and allow to marinate in the refrigerator for at least 1 hour. (For best results, marinate the beef overnight in the refrigerator.)
3. To prevent burning, soak a set of wooden skewers in cold water for 20 minutes. Place the beef and vegetables on the skewers in this order: beef–red onion–red bell pepper–yellow bell pepper. Repeat the order twice for each skewer.
4. Preheat a grill to medium heat. Place the kabobs directly on the grill and cook for about 12–14 minutes, or until the beef is done. Turn the kabobs periodically to prevent burning. When the kabobs are finished, top each with a cherry tomato and serve.

Chef's Hints: This is a great recipe for late spring, when the weather has started to warm and you want to break out the grill again. But if the day is rainy, or you just do not want to haul out the charcoal, you can also grill these kabobs using your oven broiler. Make sure you use a roasting rack so that the fat from the meat can drip away from the kabobs. Also, do not set the kabobs too close to the flames or they will burn before being fully cooked.

Stuffed Banana Peppers with Ground Beef and Pork

Ingredients

1 1/2–2 lb fresh banana peppers
1/2 lb lean ground beef
1/2 lb ground pork
1/4 cup dry bread crumbs
2 large eggs, beaten
1 tsp black pepper
1 Tbsp oregano
3 cups Spicy Marinara Sauce (see p. 148)
2 Tbsp Parmesan cheese, grated
2 Tbsp fresh parsley, chopped

4 Servings
Serving Size: about 2 peppers

Calories	400
Calories from Fat	194
Total Fat	22 g
Saturated Fat	7 g
Cholesterol	165 mg
Sodium	1408 mg
Carbohydrate	24 g
Dietary Fiber	6 g
Sugars	7 g
Protein	30 g

Exchanges
2 Other Carbohydrate
3 1/2 Lean Meat
1 Vegetable
2 Fat

Preparation

1. Preheat the oven to 350°F. Cut the tops off the banana peppers and remove the seeds. In a separate bowl, mix the beef, pork, bread crumbs, eggs, black pepper, and oregano together. Be careful not to over mix. Stuff each banana pepper with the ground meat mixture, then place the peppers in a large baking dish. Cover the peppers with the Spicy Marinara Sauce. Cover the baking dish with foil.
2. Place the dish in the oven and cook for 30 minutes, or until the peppers are tender. Serve the peppers with grated Parmesan cheese and parsley over top.

Grilled Flank Steak Teriyaki

Ingredients

- 15 oz teriyaki sauce
- 1 Tbsp brown sugar
- 1 Tbsp garlic, chopped
- 1 1/2 lb flank steak

4 Servings

Serving Size: 5 oz

Calories	288
Calories from Fat	119
Total Fat	13 g
Saturated Fat	6 g
Cholesterol	88 mg
Sodium	754 mg
Carbohydrate	4 g
Dietary Fiber	0 g
Sugars	2 g
Protein	37 g

Exchanges

5 Very Lean Meat

2 Fat

Preparation

1. Combine all the ingredients in a shallow pan and marinate, covered, for at least 1 hour in the refrigerator. (For best results, marinate the flank steak overnight in the refrigerator.)
2. Preheat the grill to medium heat. Place the flank steak directly onto the hot grill. Cook to desired doneness (8–10 minutes for rare, 10–12 minutes for medium, 12–15 minutes for well), turning the steak periodically to avoid burning.

Chef's Hints: Like the Grilled Beef Kabobs (see p. 36), this recipe can be done in an oven broiler.

*P*adre's Country Style Ribs

Ingredients

2 quarts water
1 Tbsp cinnamon
1 tsp nutmeg
1 Tbsp whole star anise
1 lb country-style pork ribs, individually cut
1 cup low-sodium soy sauce
1 cup brown sugar
1 Tbsp garlic, chopped
1 cup cider vinegar

4 Servings
Serving Size: 4.5 oz, or 1/4 of the ribs

Calories	470
Calories from Fat	309
Total Fat	34 g
Saturated Fat	13 g
Cholesterol	137 mg
Sodium	274 mg
Carbohydrate	5 g
Dietary Fiber	0 g
Sugars	4.5 g
Protein	33 g

Exchanges
5 Lean Meat
4 Fat

Preparation

1. In a large pot, bring the water to a boil. Add the cinnamon, nutmeg, star anise, and pork ribs. Bring to a boil again, then reduce the heat to a simmer. Simmer the ribs for 30 minutes, or until done.
2. Combine the remaining ingredients in a shallow dish. Remove the ribs from the water and place them in the shallow dish. Allow the ribs to marinate in the refrigerator overnight.
3. Preheat a grill or oven broiler. Place the marinated ribs on the grill or in the broiler and allow them to brown. Turn the ribs periodically until all sides are brown and fully cooked.

Grilled Marinated Pork Tenderloin

Ingredients

1/4 cup balsamic vinegar
1 Tbsp garlic, chopped
2 Tbsp olive oil
1 Tbsp fresh rosemary, minced
1 Tbsp oregano, minced
2 pork tenderloins, about 1 1/4 lb total

4 Servings
Serving Size: 4 oz

Calories	252
Calories from Fat	120
Total Fat	13 g
Saturated Fat	3 g
Cholesterol	84 mg
Sodium	61 mg
Carbohydrate	1 g
Dietary Fiber	0 g
Sugars	1 g
Protein	30 g

Exchanges
4 Very Lean Meat
2 Fat

Preparation

1. In a medium bowl, combine the balsamic vinegar and the garlic. Add the olive oil slowly while whisking to fully combine. Add the rosemary and oregano and whisk for another minute. Place the pork tenderloins in a shallow dish and pour the marinade over them. Refrigerate, covered, overnight. Turn the tenderloins periodically to allow the marinade to soak in.

2. Preheat a grill or oven broiler to medium heat. Place the tenderloins on the grill and discard the marinade. Turn the tenderloins periodically to cook fully. Cook for 20–25 minutes, or until the tenderloins reach an internal temperature of 155°F. Allow the meat to rest for 3–5 minutes before serving.

Sweet and Sour Pork over Rice

Ingredients

1 8-oz can pineapple chunks
1/4 cup brown sugar
1/4 cup cider vinegar
2 Tbsp teriyaki sauce
1/2 cup Chicken Stock (see p. 155)
1/4 cup water
2 Tbsp cornstarch
1 Tbsp sesame oil
1 cup all-purpose flour
1 Tbsp black pepper
1 lb lean boneless pork, cut into 1/2-inch strips
2 large red bell peppers, thinly sliced
2 large yellow bell peppers, thinly sliced
1 medium red onion, thinly sliced
2 Tbsp garlic, minced
1 Tbsp fresh ginger, minced
3 cups cooked white rice
1 bunch green onions, chopped

8 Servings
Serving Size: 1/2 cup sweet and sour, 1/3 cup rice

Calories	308
Calories from Fat	51
Total Fat	6 g
Saturated Fat	2 g
Cholesterol	37 mg
Sodium	208 mg
Carbohydrate	47 g
Dietary Fiber	2 g
Sugars	13 g
Protein	17 g

Exchanges
2 Starch
2 Very Lean Meat
1 Vegetable
1 Fat

Preparation

1. Drain the juice from the can of pineapple chunks into a small pot. Add the brown sugar, cider vinegar, teriyaki sauce, and chicken stock. Bring the pot to a simmer. In a separate bowl, mix the water and cornstarch until they form a smooth paste. As the liquid is simmering, whisk the cornstarch mixture into the pot to thicken the sauce. Remove the pot from the heat.

2. Heat the sesame oil in a large pan or wok over medium-high heat. Combine the flour and black pepper in a separate, shallow bowl, then dredge the pork pieces through the flour until they are coated. Add the pork to a preheated nonstick pan stirring frequently until fully cooked. Remove the pork from the pan and set aside.

3. Add the red and yellow bell peppers to the pan. Cook for 2 minutes, stirring constantly. Add the red onion to the pan and continue to stir until the onions are tender. Add the garlic and ginger. Stir for 30 seconds.

4. Return the cooked pork to the pan, then add the sweet and sour sauce from your pot. Bring the contents to a simmer for 3–4 minutes. Serve over rice and garnish with chopped green onions.

$\mathcal{B}$arbecued Chicken Wings

Ingredients

- 2 quarts water
- 2 cups cider vinegar
- 2 Tbsp garlic, minced
- 1/2 cup brown sugar
- 1 tsp black peppercorns
- 2 bay leaves
- 12 whole chicken wings
- 4 Tbsp store-bought barbecue sauce

4 Servings
Serving Size: 3 wings

Calories	308
Calories from Fat	182
Total Fat	20 g
Saturated Fat	6 g
Cholesterol	86 mg
Sodium	211 mg
Carbohydrate	2 g
Dietary Fiber	0 g
Sugars	2 g
Protein	28 g

Exchanges
4 Lean Meat
2 Fat

Preparation

1. In a large pot, combine the water, cider vinegar, garlic, brown sugar, peppercorns, and bay leaves. Bring the liquid to a simmer. Add the chicken wings and simmer for 20 minutes, or until fully cooked.
2. Preheat the grill or oven broiler. Grill the chicken wings, basting them periodically with the barbecue sauce. Be sure to turn the wings periodically to prevent burning.

Flavor Idea: For added taste when cooking on an outdoor grill, add a handful of hardwood chips to your charcoal. Many stores sell hickory or mesquite chips for barbecuing. Just be sure to soak the hardwood chips in water for an hour before you add them to the coals.

Grilled Barbecued Chicken Kabobs

Ingredients

- 5 boneless, skinless chicken breasts
- 1 large onion
- 1 green bell pepper
- 1/2 lb white mushrooms
- 1 cup store-bought barbecue sauce
- 2 oz teriyaki sauce
- 1 Tbsp honey

5 Servings
Serving Size: 2 kabobs

Calories	204
Calories from Fat	33
Total Fat	4 g
Saturated Fat	1 g
Cholesterol	78 mg
Sodium	327 mg
Carbohydrate	12 g
Dietary Fiber	2 g
Sugars	7 g
Protein	30 g

Exchanges
1/2 Other Carbohydrate
4 Very Lean Meat
1 1/2 Vegetable

Preparation

1. To prevent burning, soak a set of wooden skewers in cold water for 30 minutes. Cut the chicken, onion, green bell pepper, and mushrooms into similarly sized pieces. Place the chicken and vegetables on the skewers in this order: chicken–onion–green bell pepper–mushroom. Repeat the order twice for each skewer.
2. Combine the remaining ingredients in a shallow dish. Add the kabobs to the dish and cover them thoroughly with the liquid. Cover the dish and refrigerate for at least 30 minutes. (For best results, marinate the kabobs in the refrigerator overnight.)
3. Preheat the grill to medium heat. Preheat the oven to 325°F. Grill the kabobs on each side for 6–7 minutes. Transfer the kabobs to a roasting rack and finish them in the oven. Cook in the oven for about 20 minutes, or until the chicken is fully done.

Chicken Tenders with Roasted Garlic, Mushrooms, and Onions

Ingredients

- 1 garlic bulb
- 1 tsp olive oil
- 1 lb chicken tenders, or boneless, skinless chicken breasts cut into 3/4-inch strips
- 1 tsp salt
- 1 tsp pepper
- 1/2 cup all-purpose flour
- 1 1/2 Tbsp olive oil
- 1 medium onion, sliced
- 1/2 lb mushrooms, sliced
- 3 green onions, chopped

4 Servings

Serving Size: about 1 cup

Calories	268
Calories from Fat	99
Total Fat	11 g
Saturated Fat	2 g
Cholesterol	63 mg
Sodium	643 mg
Carbohydrate	17 g
Dietary Fiber	2 g
Sugars	4 g
Protein	26 g

Exchanges

3 Very Lean Meat
1 1/2 Vegetable
2 Fat

Preparation

1. Preheat the oven to 350°F. Slice the top of the garlic bulb so that the garlic pieces are just exposed. Place the bulb on a small baking dish and rub 1 tsp of olive oil over the skin. Put the garlic in the oven and bake for 20–30 minutes, or until the garlic bulb is soft to the touch. Remove the garlic and allow it to cool.

2. Once cool, break open the garlic bulb and squeeze the garlic pulp from the skin. Discard any of the skin or peel. Puree the roasted garlic in a food processor until it is a paste.

3. Season the chicken tenders with salt and pepper. Place the flour in a separate, shallow bowl, then dredge the chicken through the flour until it is coated. Heat 1 Tbsp of olive oil in a pan over medium-high heat. Add the chicken to the pan and cook until all sides are golden brown and the chicken is thoroughly cooked, about 8–10 minutes. Remove the chicken from the pan and set aside.

4. Add 1/2 Tbsp of olive oil to the pan and add the onions. Cook until tender, about 5 minutes. Add the mushrooms and cook for additional 3–5 minutes, or until the mushrooms are tender. Add the chicken tenders and roasted garlic puree to the pan. Stir the contents together. Serve immediately and garnish with the chopped green onions.

*L*emon Chicken with Reduced Chicken Broth

Ingredients

4 boneless, skinless chicken breasts
1 tsp salt
1/2 tsp pepper
1/2 cup all-purpose flour
2 lemons
1 Tbsp olive oil
1 Tbsp garlic, chopped
1/2 cup Chicken Stock (see p. 155)

4 Servings
Serving Size: 1 chicken breast, 2 Tbsp broth

Calories	197
Calories from Fat	58
Total Fat	7 g
Saturated Fat	1 g
Cholesterol	73 mg
Sodium	647 mg
Carbohydrate	7 g
Dietary Fiber	.5 g
Sugars	1 g
Protein	28 g

Exchanges
3 Very Lean Meat
1 Fat

Preparation

1. Season the chicken breasts with salt and pepper. Place the flour in a separate, shallow bowl, then dredge the chicken through the flour until it is coated. Using a cheese grater, grate the rind of both lemons. Squeeze the lemon juice from the two lemons into a separate bowl.
2. Heat the olive oil in a pan over medium heat. Place the chicken breasts in the pan and cook each side until it is golden brown. Add the lemon juice, grated lemon rind, and garlic to the pan. Continue cooking until the pan is almost dry again, turning the chicken once while cooking.
3. Add the chicken stock to the pan and bring the liquid to a simmer. Cook until the liquid has been reduced by half. Serve chicken breasts with reduced liquid on top.

*T*arragon Chicken

Ingredients

4 boneless chicken breasts, with skin
4 sprigs fresh tarragon
1 tsp salt
2 tsp pepper
1 Tbsp olive oil

4 Servings
Serving Size: 1 chicken breast

Calories	234
Calories from Fat	102
Total Fat	11 g
Saturated Fat	3 g
Cholesterol	86 mg
Sodium	654 mg
Carbohydrate	1 g
Dietary Fiber	0 g
Sugars	0 g
Protein	31 g

Exchanges
4 Very Lean Meat
2 Fat

Preparation

1. Preheat the oven to 375°F. Gently lift the skin of each chicken breast and place a sprig of tarragon underneath. Season each chicken breast with salt and pepper.
2. Heat the olive oil in a pan over medium heat. Add the chicken breasts and cook each side until it is golden brown.
3. Remove the chicken breasts to a baking sheet. Place the breasts in the oven and cook for about 20 minutes, or until the chicken has reached an internal temperature of 165°F. Remove the chicken from the oven and allow it to rest for 5 minutes before serving.

Chef's Hints: When searing the chicken, sear the breast with the skin on. By doing this you will protect the meat from burning and retain some of the juices. Remove the skin before serving.

Grilled Turkey Breast

Ingredients

1/4 cup cider vinegar
1/2 Tbsp garlic, minced
  1 Tbsp ground mustard
  1 Tbsp honey
1/2 Tbsp brown sugar
1/2 tsp black pepper
1/2 cup olive oil
  4 turkey cutlets

4 Servings
Serving Size: 1 cutlet

Calories	176
Calories from Fat	9
Total Fat	1 g
Saturated Fat	0 g
Cholesterol	20 mg
Sodium	88 mg
Carbohydrate	1 g
Dietary Fiber	0 g
Sugars	1 g
Protein	9 g

Exchanges
3 Very Lean Meat

Preparation

1. In a medium bowl, combine the cider vinegar, garlic, ground mustard, honey, brown sugar, and black pepper. Slowly whisk in the olive oil to thoroughly combine.
2. Place the turkey cutlets in a shallow dish and pour the liquid over top. Cover and place in the refrigerator for at least 1 hour. (For best results, marinate overnight in the refrigerator.)
3. Preheat the grill or oven broiler. Place the breasts directly on the grill, or on a roasting rack beneath the broiler. Cook for about 20–25 minutes, or until the turkey is fully done. Turn the breasts frequently to prevent burning.

Greek Pasta Salad

Ingredients

3 Tbsp balsamic vinegar
1/3 cup extra virgin olive oil
3/4 tsp garlic, minced
3/4 tsp fresh oregano, chopped
3/4 tsp fresh mint, chopped
1/4 tsp black pepper
1/2 lb orechetta pasta (or the pasta of your choice), cooked and cooled
12 cherry tomatoes, cut into quarters
1/2 small red onion, sliced
1/2 cucumber, diced
1 red bell pepper, sliced
1/4 cup pitted Greek olives

6 Servings
Serving Size: about 1 cup

Calories	429
Calories from Fat	263
Total Fat	29 g
Saturated Fat	4 g
Cholesterol	0 mg
Sodium	100 mg
Carbohydrate	37 g
Dietary Fiber	2.5 g
Sugars	4 g
Protein	6 g

Exchanges
2 Starch
1/2 Vegetable
5 1/2 Fat

Preparation

1. In a small bowl, add the balsamic vinegar. Whisk the olive oil in slowly until it is thoroughly combined. Add the garlic, oregano, mint, and black pepper.
2. In a separate bowl, combine the cooled pasta with the remaining ingredients. Pour the vinaigrette over the pasta and toss until well-coated. Refrigerate for 1 hour before serving.

Pizza with Plum Tomato and Basil

Ingredients

1 Tbsp olive oil
1 premade pizza pie shell
1 cup Spicy Marinara
   Sauce (see p. 148)
1 cup low-fat mozzarella
   cheese, grated
6 leaves fresh basil, very
   thinly cut
3 plum tomatoes, thinly
   sliced

6 Servings
Serving Size: 1 slice

Calories	244
Calories from Fat	101
Total Fat	11 g
Saturated Fat	5 g
Cholesterol	20 mg
Sodium	772 mg
Carbohydrate	23 g
Dietary Fiber	3 g
Sugars	7 g
Protein	14 g

Exchanges
2 Starch
1 1/2 Lean Meat
1/2 Vegetable
1 Fat

Preparation

1. Preheat the oven to 425°F. If you are using a baking sheet, coat it with the olive oil. (If you have a pizza stone, you can eliminate the olive oil. Simply place the stone in the oven to preheat it.)
2. Cover the top of the pizza pie shell with the Spicy Marinara Sauce. Sprinkle the cheese over the top so that it covers the sauce evenly. Sprinkle the basil evenly overtop. Place the plum tomatoes around the pizza.
3. Place the pizza in the oven (on a stone or baking sheet) and cook for 12–15 minutes, or until the pizza dough is firm and lightly browned. Remove from the oven and allow it to cool for 3 minutes before serving.

Did You Know? The tomato is classified as a fruit, not a vegetable. It also happens to be one of the most nutritious fruits around.

Crab Cakes

Ingredients

- 1 large egg
- 1/2 cup fresh bread crumbs
- 1 tsp black pepper
- 2 green onions, minced
- 1 Tbsp Dijon mustard
- 1 lb lump crab meat
- Nonstick cooking spray

4 Servings
Serving Size: 1 crab cake

Calories	235
Calories from Fat	86
Total Fat	10 g
Saturated Fat	2 g
Cholesterol	159 mg
Sodium	840 mg
Carbohydrate	11 g
Dietary Fiber	1 g
Sugars	>1 g
Protein	25 g

Exchanges
1 Starch
3 1/2 Very Lean Meat
1 1/2 Fat

Preparation

1. Preheat the oven to 350°F. In a medium bowl, beat the egg. Add the bread crumbs, black pepper, green onions, and mustard. Mix well. Gently mix in the crab meat until the mixture binds together.
2. Spray a baking dish with the nonstick cooking spray. Shape the crab mixture into 4 patties and place them in the baking dish. Bake the patties for 18–20 minutes.

Grilled Halibut with Pineapple

Ingredients

4 halibut steaks, 1/2-inch thick
1 tsp salt
1 tsp white pepper
2 Tbsp lemon juice
1 small pineapple
2 Tbsp fresh chives, chopped

4 Servings
Serving Size: 1 halibut steak, 1 pineapple slice

Calories	348
Calories from Fat	196
Total Fat	22 g
Saturated Fat	4 g
Cholesterol	71 mg
Sodium	706 mg
Carbohydrate	16 g
Dietary Fiber	2 g
Sugars	14 g
Protein	23 g

Exchanges
3 1/2 Very Lean Meat
1 Fruit
4 Fat

Preparation

1. Preheat the grill or oven broiler. Season the halibut with salt and pepper. Baste one side with the lemon juice. Place the halibut steaks on the grill or on a roasting rack beneath the broiler. When the halibut becomes white in color and firm to the touch, turn the steaks over and baste the remaining side with lemon juice. Cook until the entire fish is firm and flaky.
2. Trim the pineapple, remove its core, and cut the rest into 4 slices. Grill the pineapple or place it under a broiler until it is tender, about 5 minutes. Serve the halibut with the pineapple on top and garnish with the chives.

Grilled Shrimp over Herb Basmati Rice with Asparagus and Baby Carrots

Ingredients

1	Tbsp olive oil
1	Tbsp garlic, chopped
1	cup basmati rice
1	Tbsp fresh thyme, chopped
1	Tbsp fresh oregano, chopped
1	Tbsp fresh chives, chopped
2	cups water
1	quart water
2	tsp sugar
1	tsp white vinegar
1/2	lb baby carrots
1	cup water
1/2	tsp salt
1/2	lb asparagus, washed and trimmed
1	lemon wedge
1	lb large shrimp, deveined and without shells
1	tsp red pepper flakes
1	Tbsp olive oil

4 Servings

Serving Size: 1/4 lb shrimp, 1/2 cup vegetables, 3/4 cup rice

Calories	370
Calories from Fat	79
Total Fat	9 g
Saturated Fat	1 g
Cholesterol	161 mg
Sodium	212 mg
Carbohydrate	50 g
Dietary Fiber	2 g
Sugars	4 g
Protein	24 g

Exchanges

2 Starch
2 1/2 Very Lean Meat
1 1/2 Vegetable
1 Fat

Preparation

1. Preheat a grill or oven broiler. To prevent burning, soak a set of wooden skewers in cold water for 30 minutes.
2. Heat 1 Tbsp of olive oil in a medium pot over medium heat. Add the garlic and stir quickly for 30 seconds, or until the garlic turns white in color. Add the basmati rice and continue to stir until the rice is well coated. Add the thyme, oregano, chives, and water. Bring the liquid to a simmer. Cover and cook for 15 minutes.
3. Fill a separate pot with water and bring it to a boil. Add the sugar, vinegar, and baby carrots. Bring the liquid to a simmer. Cook the baby carrots for 10 minutes, or until tender.
4. While the baby carrots are cooking, steam the asparagus. Place 1 cup of water in a large pan and bring it to a boil. Add the salt and asparagus. Cover the pan and allow the asparagus to steam for 3–4 minutes, or until it is bright green but still firm. Drain the water and season the asparagus with juice from the lemon wedge.
5. Season the shrimp with the red pepper flakes. Place the shrimp on the wooden skewers, brush the skewers with olive oil, and arrange them on the grill or beneath a broiler. Cook the shrimp for 2 minutes, then turn the shrimp over and cook the remaining side for 2 minutes. The shrimp are done when they are firm to the touch and pinkish in color.
6. Serve the shrimp and vegetables over the basmati rice.

Chef's Hints: If your asparagus becomes limp, revive it by placing it in ice cold water for approximately 45 seconds before cooking.

Pan-Seared Flounder Almondine

Ingredients

- 1/2 cup almonds, crushed or sliced
- 4 flounder filets, 6 oz each
- 1/2 tsp salt
- 1/4 tsp black pepper
- 1 cup reduced fat (2%) milk
- 1 cup all-purpose flour
  Nonstick cooking spray
- 1 lemon, cut into wedges

4 Servings
Serving Size: 1 filet

Calories	227
Calories from Fat	32
Total Fat	4 g
Saturated Fat	1 g
Cholesterol	124 mg
Sodium	190 mg
Carbohydrate	4 g
Dietary Fiber	0 g
Sugars	1 g
Protein	43 g

Exchanges
6 Very Lean Meat

Preparation

1. Preheat the oven to 350°F. When the oven has heated, place the almonds on a baking sheet and bake until they are lightly browned, about 8–10 minutes. Remove from the oven and cool.
2. Season the flounder with salt and pepper. Dip the filet into the milk, then dredge it through the flour.
3. Spray a pan with nonstick cooking spray and heat it over medium heat. Place the filets in the pan. Lightly brown one side, then turn the filets to brown the other side. When the filets are done, serve with a lemon wedge and a garnish of the toasted almonds.

South Carolina Soft-Shell Crab

Ingredients

4   soft-shell crabs
1   tsp black pepper
1   tsp red pepper flakes
1   tsp garlic powder
1/2 cup all-purpose flour
2   Tbsp olive oil

4 Servings
Serving Size: 1 crab

Calories	189
Calories from Fat	54
Total Fat	6 g
Saturated Fat	.5 g
Cholesterol	122 mg
Sodium	433 mg
Carbohydrate	3 g
Dietary Fiber	0 g
Sugars	0 g
Protein	28 g

Exchanges
4 Very Lean Meat
1 Fat

Preparation

1. Turn the crab upside down. Peel back the undershell and remove the top shell. Remove the long gills and the lungs. Remove any excess innards. Wash the crabs under cold, running water. Pat dry.
2. Season the crabs with black pepper, red pepper flakes, and garlic powder. Place the flour in a separate, shallow bowl, then dredge the crabs through the flour until coated.
3. Heat the olive oil in a pan over medium heat. Place the crabs in the pan, brown them on one side, then turn the crabs over and repeat. When the crabs are fully cooked, pat them dry with a paper towel and serve immediately.

Gazpacho Soup

Ingredients

- 1 lb plum tomatoes, peeled and seeded
- 1 cup cucumber, peeled, seeded, and diced
- 1/2 jalapeño pepper, seeded, diced
- 1/2 medium red onion, diced
- 1/4 bunch cilantro, chopped
- 1 4.5-oz can of tomato juice
- 1/2 tsp hot pepper sauce
- 1/4 tsp salt

4 Servings
Serving Size: 1 cup

Calories	49
Calories from Fat	5
Total Fat	1 g
Saturated Fat	0 g
Cholesterol	0 mg
Sodium	272 mg
Carbohydrate	11 g
Dietary Fiber	3 g
Sugars	5 g
Protein	2 g

Exchanges
2 Vegetables

Preparation

1. Combine all ingredients in a food processor and blend until smooth. Add more salt if needed. Refrigerate for 1 hour before serving.

Grilled Apple Pear Soup

Ingredients

- 2 medium Granny Smith apples, peeled and halved
- 2 medium Bosc pears, peeled and halved
- 2 medium Red Delicious apples, peeled and halved
- 1/2 cup shallots, chopped
- 1 cup Apple Jack liquor
- 1/3 cup cider vinegar
- 1/2 cup Chicken Stock (see p. 155)
- 1 Tbsp brown sugar
  Pinch salt
  Pinch white pepper
- 2–3 Tbsp whipped cream
  Pinch cinnamon

6 Servings
Serving Size: about 1 cup

Calories	178
Calories from Fat	4
Total Fat	>1 g
Saturated Fat	0 g
Cholesterol	0 mg
Sodium	8 mg
Carbohydrate	36 g
Dietary Fiber	4 g
Sugars	27 g
Protein	1 g

Exchanges
1 1/2 Fruit
1/2 Vegetable

Preparation

1. Preheat the oven broiler. Place apple and pear halves beneath the broiler and allow them to brown. Turn the halves over and brown the remaining side. Remove them from the broiler. When the apples cool, peel and remove seeds. Dice apples and pears into 1/2-inch pieces.
2. In a large pot over medium-high, add the shallot and the Apple Jack liquor. Bring it to a simmer and allow the liquid to reduce by half. Add the grilled apples and pears, cider vinegar, chicken stock, and brown sugar. Bring the liquid back to a simmer. Cook about 35–45 minutes, or until the apples and pears are very tender.
3. Remove the mixture from the heat and allow it to cool slightly. Place the contents into a food processor and blend until smooth. Add the salt and white pepper.
4. Serve immediately with 1 Tbsp of whipped cream and a pinch cinnamon as a garnish.

Spinach, Red Onion, and Cherry Tomato Salad with Tarragon Vinaigrette

Ingredients

1/3 cup rice wine vinegar
2/3 cup olive oil
1 shallot, minced
1/4 cup fresh tarragon, minced
1/2 tsp salt
Pinch black pepper
3/4 lb spinach
1/2 pint cherry tomatoes, cut into quarters
1/2 red onion, thinly sliced
4 oz Roquefort blue cheese

4 Servings

Serving Size: 1/4 of salad, 1 Tbsp dressing

Calories	216
Calories from Fat	162
Total Fat	18 g
Saturated Fat	7 g
Cholesterol	26 mg
Sodium	645 mg
Carbohydrate	7 g
Dietary Fiber	3 g
Sugars	2 g
Protein	9 g

Exchanges

1 Lean Meat
1 Vegetable
3 Fat

Preparation

1. In a medium bowl, add the vinegar. Slowly whisk in the olive oil until it is thoroughly mixed. Add the shallot, tarragon, salt, and black pepper. Mix well.
2. Rinse the spinach beneath cold, running water, then pat dry. Remove the stems, then coarsely chop the spinach.
3. Place the spinach in the center of the plate. Arrange the quartered tomatoes around the edges. Place the onions over the top of the spinach, then drizzle the salad with 1 Tbsp of the tarragon dressing. Crumble 1 oz of the cheese on top and serve.

Chef's Hints: To keep your salad from becoming soggy, place a saucer upside down in the bottom of the salad bowl. The water will drain off the saucer and leave the salad dry.

Corn Salsa

Ingredients

- 1/3 lb frozen corn kernels
- 1/3 cup red bell pepper, diced
- 1/3 cup yellow bell pepper, diced
- 2/3 cup cherry tomatoes, sliced into quarters
- 1/4 cup red onion, diced
- 1/2 small cucumber, peeled and diced
- 1/2 jalapeño pepper, seeded and minced
- 1 tsp garlic, minced
- 2 tsp fresh cilantro, chopped
- 1/3 tsp salt
- 1/3 tsp black pepper

4 Servings
Serving Size: 1/2 cup

Calories	51
Calories from Fat	3
Total Fat	>1 g
Saturated Fat	0 g
Cholesterol	0 mg
Sodium	199 mg
Carbohydrate	12 g
Dietary Fiber	2 g
Sugars	2 g
Protein	2 g

Exchanges
1/2 Starch
1 Vegetable

Preparation

1. In a medium pot, bring water to a boil. Add the corn kernels and cook for 5 minutes. Drain the water and allow the corn to cool.
2. Combine the corn and all the remaining ingredients into a bowl and mix well. Refrigerate for 1 hour before serving.

Grilled Portabello Mushrooms

Ingredients

1 Tbsp garlic, minced
2 tsp fresh rosemary, minced
2 Tbsp olive oil
2 Tbsp balsamic vinegar
2 Portabello mushroom caps

4 Servings
Serving Size: 1/2
  Portabello cap

Calories	86
Calories from Fat	61
Total Fat	6 g
Saturated Fat	0 g
Cholesterol	0 mg
Sodium	9 mg
Carbohydrate	6 g
Dietary Fiber	2 g
Sugars	1 g
Protein	2 g

Exchanges
1/2 Vegetable
1 Fat

Preparation

1. In a small bowl, combine the garlic, rosemary, olive oil, and vinegar. Mix well. Using a pastry brush, cover both sides of the Portabello mushrooms with the mixture. Cover and refrigerate for 30 minutes.
2. Preheat the grill or oven broiler. Grill the mushrooms on low heat, or place them on a rack that is low in the oven. Cook each side of the Portabello for 5 minutes. Serve immediately.

Did You Know? You can keep your vegetables crisp by placing a few sponges at the bottom of your vegetable drawer. The sponges will absorb the moisture.

Grilled Herbed Zucchini Halves

Ingredients

- 1/4 cup red wine vinegar
- 2 Tbsp shallots, chopped
- 3/4 cup extra virgin olive oil
- 2 tsp lemon rind, grated
- 1 Tbsp fresh thyme, chopped
- 1 Tbsp fresh oregano, chopped
- 1 tsp fresh rosemary, chopped
- 1 tsp fresh mint, chopped
- 2 quarts water
- 1 tsp salt
- 2 small zucchini

4 Servings
Serving Size: 1/2 zucchini

Calories	110
Calories from Fat	84
Total Fat	9 g
Saturated Fat	1 g
Cholesterol	0 mg
Sodium	6 mg
Carbohydrate	6 g
Dietary Fiber	2.5 g
Sugars	3 g
Protein	2 g

Exchanges
1/2 Vegetable
2 Fat

Preparation

1. In a medium bowl, add the red wine vinegar and the shallots. Slowly whisk in the olive oil until it is thoroughly combined. Add the lemon rind, thyme, oregano, rosemary, and mint. Mix well.
2. In a pot, bring the water to a boil. Add the salt and the zucchini and simmer for 1 minute. Remove the zucchini from the water and allow it to cool. Slice the zucchini in half lengthwise. Coat the zucchini with the vinaigrette mixture. Cover and refrigerate for 1 hour.
3. Preheat the grill or an oven broiler. Set the zucchini on the grill or beneath the broiler. You are only trying to reheat the zucchini, so do not let them stay on the grill or in the broiler for more than 3–5 minutes. Serve immediately.

Grilled Marinated Potatoes

Ingredients

3	quarts water
1	Tbsp salt
1 1/2	lb red potatoes
3/4	cup low-fat Italian dressing
1/2	tsp black pepper

6 Servings
Serving Size: about 1/2 cup

Calories	176
Calories from Fat	14
Total Fat	2 g
Saturated Fat	0 g
Cholesterol	0 mg
Sodium	189 mg
Carbohydrate	37 g
Dietary Fiber	3 g
Sugars	3 g
Protein	4 g

Exchanges
2 Starch

Preparation

1. In a large pot, bring the water to a boil. Add the salt and the red potatoes. Bring the water to a simmer and cook for 12–15 minutes, until the potatoes are almost done. Remove the potatoes from the water and allow them to cool for 10 minutes.
2. Slice the potatoes into 1/2-inch thick coins and place them in a shallow dish. Pour the Italian dressing over them. Cover and refrigerate for at least 1 hour. (For more flavor, let the potatoes marinate overnight.)
3. Preheat the grill or oven broiler. Place the potatoes on the grill or beneath the broiler. Cook the potatoes until golden brown, about 8–10 minutes. To prevent burning, turn the potatoes every minute or two. Season with black pepper and serve.

Red Potato Salad

Ingredients

2   quarts water
1   lb red potatoes
6   Tbsp red onions, diced
1/2 cup celery, diced
3   Tbsp light mayonnaise
2   Tbsp Dijon mustard
1/2 tsp salt
1/2 tsp black pepper
2   green onions, chopped

---

6 Servings
Serving Size: 1/2 cup

Calories	110
Calories from Fat	28
Total Fat	3 g
Saturated Fat	0 g
Cholesterol	3 mg
Sodium	587 mg
Carbohydrate	20 g
Dietary Fiber	2 g
Sugars	3 g
Protein	2

Exchanges
1 Starch
1/2 Vegetable
1/2 Fat

Preparation

1. In a large pot, bring the water to a boil. Add the potatoes. Return the water to a simmer, cover, and cook for 15–20 minutes, or until the potatoes are done. Remove the potatoes from the water and let them cool.
2. Cut the potatoes into quarters and place them in a large bowl. Add the next six ingredients and mix together gently. Refrigerate overnight. Garnish with chopped green onions.

Spanish Rice

Ingredients

- 1 tsp olive oil
- 1/2 cup onion, diced
- 1/2 cup red bell peppers, diced
- 1/2 cup green bell peppers, diced
- 2 tsp jalapeño pepper, finely diced
- 1 Tbsp garlic, chopped
- 1 10-oz can tomatoes, diced
- 3 cups Chicken Stock (see p. 155)
- 2 tsp cumin
- 2 cups basmati rice
- 1/2 cup green onions, chopped
- 2 tsp fresh oregano, chopped
- 2 tsp fresh cilantro, chopped
- 1 tsp salt
- 1/4 tsp black pepper

6 Servings
Serving Size: 2/3 cup

Calories	291
Calories from Fat	18
Total Fat	2 g
Saturated Fat	0 g
Cholesterol	0 mg
Sodium	462 mg
Carbohydrate	63 g
Dietary Fiber	2 g
Sugars	4 g
Protein	7 g

Exchanges
3 Starch
1 1/2 Vegetable

Preparation

1. Heat the olive oil a large pot over medium heat. Add the onion, red bell pepper, green bell pepper, jalapeño, and garlic. Cook until the onion is translucent, or about 4 minutes. Add the tomatoes, chicken stock, cumin, and rice. Stir gently. Bring the liquid to a boil, reduce the heat to low, and simmer for 15–20 minutes.
2. When the rice is finished, add the remaining ingredients and mix well. Serve immediately.

Blackberry Cobbler

Ingredients

1/4 cup water
2 Tbsp sugar
1 tsp vanilla extract
1 Tbsp orange rind, grated
4 cups fresh or frozen blackberries
3 Tbsp cornstarch
3 Tbsp water
1 Pie Pastry (see p. 151)
2 Tbsp butter, melted

4 Servings
Serving Size: 1 cobbler

Calories	412
Calories from Fat	132
Total Fat	15 g
Saturated Fat	1 g
Cholesterol	0 mg
Sodium	77 mg
Carbohydrate	66 g
Dietary Fiber	9 g
Sugars	23 g
Protein	5 g

Exchanges
3 Other Carbohydrate
1 Fruit
3 Fat

Preparation

1. Preheat the oven to 350°F. In a medium pot, combine the 1/4 cup water, sugar, vanilla extract, and orange rind. Bring the liquid to a boil. Add the blackberries and lower the heat to medium-high. Stir gently, allowing the blackberries to cook and burst.
2. In a separate bowl, combine the cornstarch and the water until they form a smooth paste. Pour the cornstarch mixture into the pot and stir, letting the liquid thicken. Pour the liquid into 4 individual, oven-proof dishes.
3. Roll out the pie pastry and cut it into 4 equal pieces. Cover the top of each baking dish with a piece of pastry. Using a pastry brush, brush the tops of the pastry with butter. Put all the dishes into the oven and bake for 35 minutes, or until the pastry top is golden brown. Remove from the oven and let cool for 10 minutes.

*L*ime and Mint Granita

Ingredients

  2 cups water
  1 Tbsp fresh mint leaves
1/3 cup sugar
  3 limes, juiced

4 Servings
Serving Size: about 1/2 cup

Calories	90
Calories from Fat	0
Total Fat	0 g
Saturated Fat	0 g
Cholesterol	0 mg
Sodium	5 mg
Carbohydrate	24 g
Dietary Fiber	0 g
Sugars	22 g
Protein	0 g

Exchanges
1 1/2 Other Carbohydrate

Preparation

1. Bring the water to a simmer and add the mint leaves. Let the mint leaves simmer for 10–12 minutes. Strain the liquid onto the sugar. Mix well. Add the lime juice and allow the mixture to cool.
2. Place the mixture into the freezer. Check the mixture every hour and stir it to combine the frozen and unfrozen ingredients. The end product will be a soft frozen ice and will take 5–7 hours.

*F*resh Apple-Pear Chutney

Ingredients

- 1 medium Red Delicious apple, peeled
- 1 Granny Smith apple, peeled
- 1 medium Bartlett pear
- 1/2 cup raisins
- 1 Tbsp orange rind, grated
- 1/4 cup orange juice
- 1/4 tsp vanilla extract
- 1/4 tsp cinnamon
- 5 fresh mint leaves, finely chopped

8 Servings
Serving Size: 1/8 recipe

Calories	67
Calories from Fat	0
Total Fat	0 g
Saturated Fat	0 g
Cholesterol	0 mg
Sodium	1 mg
Carbohydrate	17 g
Dietary Fiber	2 g
Sugars	14 g
Protein	1 g

Exchanges
1 Fruit

Preparation

1. Core the apples and the pear. Dice the apples and the pear into 1/2-inch cubes and place them in a medium bowl. Add the rest of the ingredients and mix well. Cover and refrigerate for about 3 hours. Serve chilled

*V*anilla-Chocolate Parfette

Ingredients

- 1 pkg. sugar-free vanilla pudding mix
- 1 pkg. sugar-free chocolate pudding mix
- 16 individual graham squares (or 1/2 cup crumbs)
- 2 oz semi-sweet chocolate, grated
- 1/2 cup fat-free whipped topping (optional)

4 Servings
Serving Size: 1 parfette

Calories	135
Calories from Fat	44
Total Fat	5 g
Saturated Fat	3 g
Cholesterol	1 mg
Sodium	137 mg
Carbohydrate	22 g
Dietary Fiber	1 g
Sugars	13 g
Protein	2 g

Exchanges
1 1/2 Other Carbohydrate
1/2 Fat

Preparation

1. In separate bowls, prepare the vanilla and chocolate pudding mixes according to the package directions. Cover and refrigerate both puddings.
2. Crush the graham crackers into crumbs. Layer the parfette into 4 small custard cups, parfait glasses, or wine glasses. Spread 1 Tbsp chocolate pudding per serving. Top with 1 Tbsp graham cracker crumbs. Top with 1 Tbsp vanilla pudding. Top with 1 tablespoon graham cracker crumbs. Repeat for a second layer.
3. Garnish with the grated chocolate. Add a dollop of fat-free whipped topping if you wish. Serve.

Fall

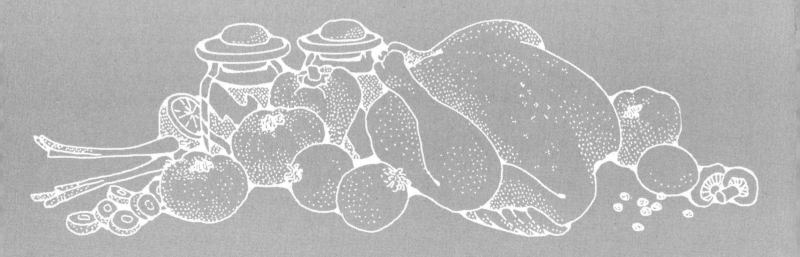

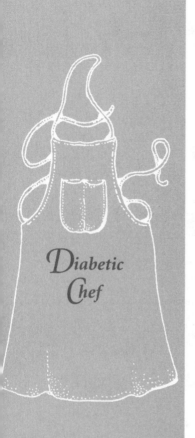

Diabetic Chef

Fall is my favorite time of the year. Change is in the air as the temperature cools and the leaves on the trees cascade with vibrant reds, yellows, and browns. The land is preparing for the long winter months, but it shares with us its last joyous expression of beauty before it heads for quiet slumber.

Fall is also the season of bounty. This is the time when many fruits and vegetables are harvested and sent directly to markets or displayed on roadside stands. Some of my fondest childhood memories are of spending the day driving to those stands and shopping.

Each October, friends and family would meet on a Saturday and drive through the farmland of eastern Long Island. Four or five cars would carry the 20 or so parents, children, and friends to a variety of farm stands and open fields. There we would either shop for, or perhaps go out to pick our own, vegetables. It was an all day trip, but nothing could have been more fun.

With fall in mind, I have selected a number of recipes that best suit the changing season. Some highlights include a hearty *Lentil Soup*, which is simple but full of flavor. The *Broiled Lamb Chops with Onion Confit* can be a dish for two or for a dinner party. It combines the complex flavors of carmelized onions with balsamic vinegar. Finally, try the *Crepes Stuffed with Bosc Pears Poached in Cabernet Sauvignon*. Bosc pears are at their peak freshness now, and this recipe puts them to excellent use.

$\mathcal{E}$gg Burritos

Ingredients

- 1 tsp butter
- 1/4 cup red bell pepper, diced
- 1/4 cup green bell pepper, diced
- 1/4 cup red onion, diced
- 1 Tbsp black olives, chopped
- 8 large eggs, beaten
- 4 10-inch flour tortilla shells
- 1/4 cup cheddar cheese, grated
- 1/4 cup salsa
- 1 tsp fresh cilantro, chopped

4 Servings
Serving Size: 1 burrito

Calories	433
Calories from Fat	168
Total Fat	19 g
Saturated Fat	7 g
Cholesterol	435 mg
Sodium	533 mg
Carbohydrate	44 g
Dietary Fiber	3 g
Sugars	4 g
Protein	21 g

Exchanges
3 Starch
2 Lean Meat
1/2 Vegetable
2 Fat

Preparation

1. Melt the butter in a pan over medium heat. And the red and green bell peppers, onion, and olives. Cook until the vegetables are tender, about 4–5 minutes. Add the beaten eggs to the pan and stir until the eggs are fully cooked.
2. Meanwhile, heat the tortilla shells in either the microwave or the oven. Spoon 1/4 of the cooked egg mixture onto each tortilla. Top with cheese, salsa, and cilantro. Serve.

Egg White Omelet with Mushrooms, Peppers, and Herbs

Ingredients

2 tsp butter
1/2 lb mushrooms, sliced
1 red bell pepper, diced
1 yellow bell pepper, diced
2 sprigs fresh thyme, leaves removed and chopped
2 sprigs fresh oregano, leaves removed and chopped
1 bunch fresh chives, chopped
  Nonstick cooking spray
8 large eggs
1 Tbsp water

4 Servings
Serving Size: 1 omelet

Calories	80
Calories from Fat	21
Total Fat	2 g
Saturated Fat	1 g
Cholesterol	5 mg
Sodium	215 mg
Carbohydrate	7 g
Dietary Fiber	2 g
Sugars	3 g
Protein	9 g

Exchanges

1 1/2 Very Lean Meat
1 Vegetable
1/2 Fat

Preparation

1. Melt 1 tsp of the butter in a pan over medium heat. Add the mushrooms and cook for 4–5 minutes, or until slightly brown. Remove the mushrooms and set aside.
2. Melt another teaspoon of butter in the pan. Add the red and yellow bell peppers. Cook until tender, about 4–5 minutes. Remove the peppers and set aside. Combine the chopped herbs in a bowl and mix.
3. For each omelet, crack two eggs into a bowl and remove the yolks. Add 1 1/2 tsp of water for every two eggs and mix well. Spray a pan with nonstick cooking spray and heat over medium heat. Pour the two egg whites into the pan. Using a wooden spoon, carefully push the edge of the egg whites toward the middle of the pan and allow the raw egg white to spread outward.
4. When the egg white begins to firm, add 1/4 of the cooked mushrooms and peppers and 2 tsp of the mixed herbs. Gently press the ingredients into the egg whites. Carefully roll the egg white so that you can turn it over and cook the other side for about 30 seconds. Remove the omelet to a plate and serve.

Chopped Steak with Pepper Gravy

Ingredients

- 4 4-oz pieces chopped steak (also called minute or cubed steak)
- 1 tsp salt
- 1/2 tsp black pepper
- 1/4 cup all-purpose flour
- 1 Tbsp olive oil
- 1 cup evaporated skim milk
- 1 tsp black pepper
- 2 Tbsp cornstarch
- 2 Tbsp water
- 2 Tbsp fresh parsley, chopped

4 Servings
Serving Size: 1 steak, 1/4 cup gravy

Calories	482
Calories from Fat	335
Total Fat	37 g
Saturated Fat	14 g
Cholesterol	87 mg
Sodium	712 mg
Carbohydrate	13 g
Dietary Fiber	.5 g
Sugars	7 g
Protein	23 g

Exchanges
1/2 Starch
2 1/2 Lean Meat
6 Fat

Preparation

1. Season the steak with salt and pepper. Place the flour in a separate, shallow bowl, then dredge the steak through it until the steak is covered. Heat the olive oil in a pan over medium-high heat. Add the steak to the pan. Cook for 5–8 minutes, turning once to brown both sides. Remove the steak from the pan and keep it warm.
2. Put the evaporated skim milk and black pepper in a medium sauce pot and bring it to a simmer. In a separate bowl, mix the cornstarch and water until it forms a smooth paste. Whisk the cornstarch slowly into the pot until the gravy thickens.
3. Serve the chopped steak topped with the pepper gravy and garnish with the chopped parsley.

Chef's Hints: Cornstarch is the ideal thickener for sauces, gravies, and soups. If you are not careful, though, you could form lumps while trying to thicken your liquid. Be sure to add your water and cornstarch solution slowly to avoid lumps.

*M*eat Loaf

Ingredients

1 lb lean ground beef
1/2 cup onion, diced
1/2 cup green bell pepper, diced
1/4 tsp black pepper
1 tsp garlic powder
1/4 cup low-fat (1%) milk
1 large egg, beaten
1 tsp oregano
1 tsp thyme
1 Tbsp catsup

5 Servings
Serving Size: 5 oz

Calories	208
Calories from Fat	95
Total Fat	11 g
Saturated Fat	4 g
Cholesterol	119 mg
Sodium	171 mg
Carbohydrate	5 g
Dietary Fiber	1 g
Sugars	2 g
Protein	22 g

Exchanges
3 Lean Meat
1/2 Fat

Preparation

1. Preheat the oven to 350°F. Combine all the ingredients except the catsup and mix until just incorporated. Mold the mixture into a loaf and place it on a baking sheet. Bake in the oven for 20–25 minutes. Top the meat loaf with catsup and return it to the oven for 5 more minutes.

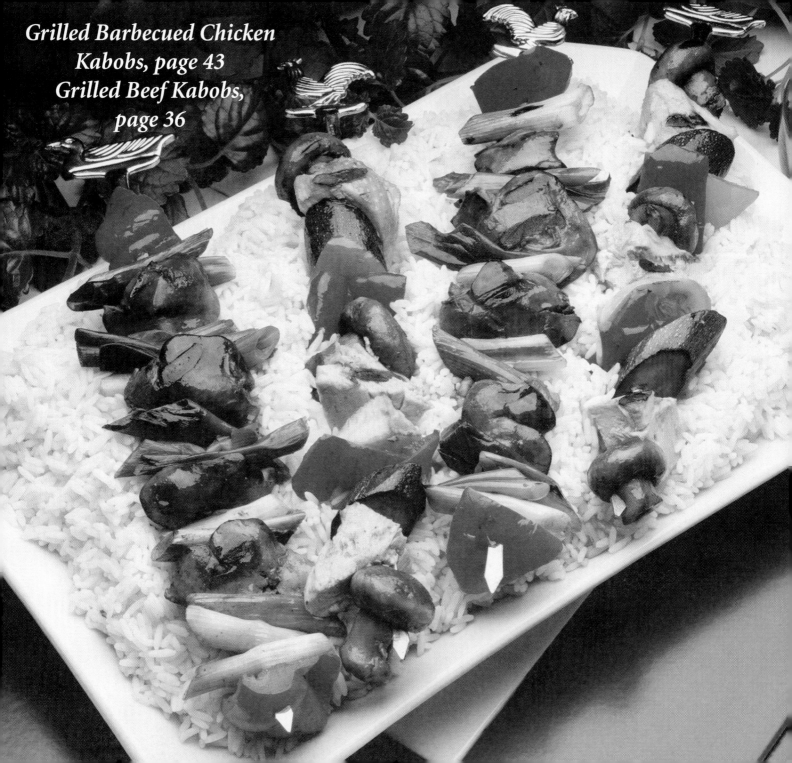

Grilled Barbecued Chicken Kabobs, page 43
Grilled Beef Kabobs, page 36

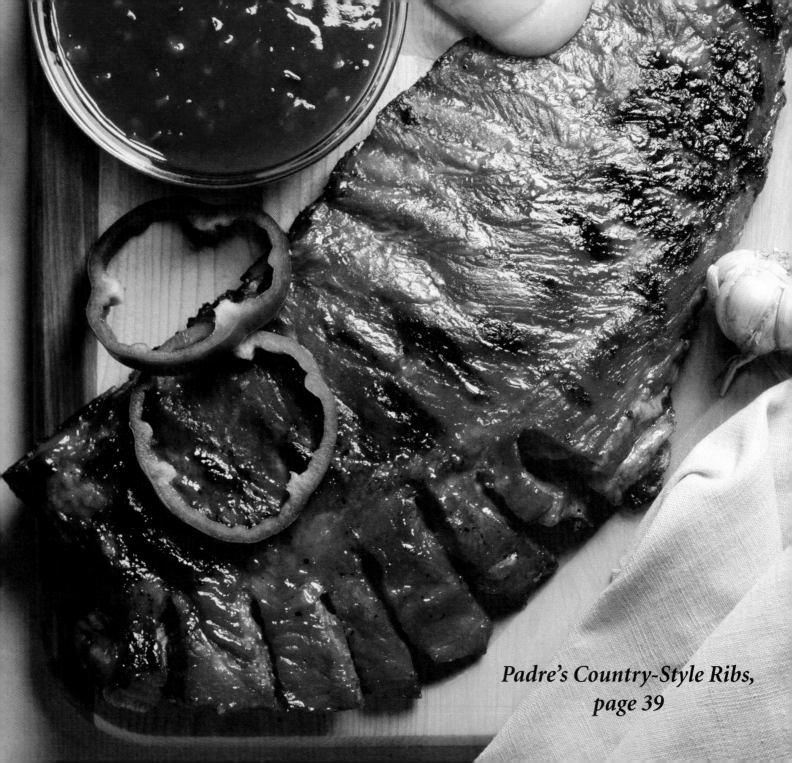

Padre's Country-Style Ribs,
page 39

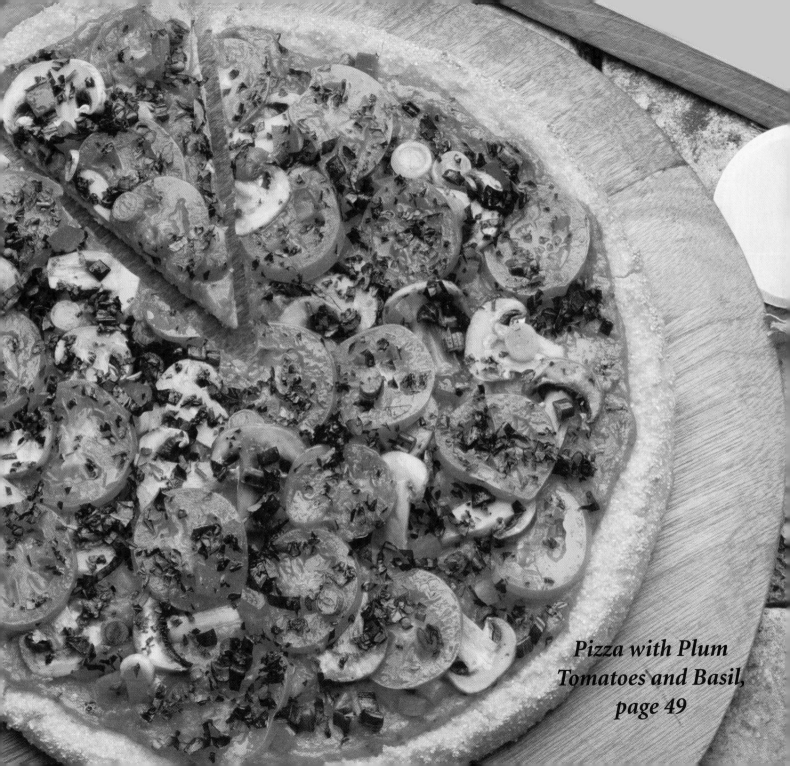

Pizza with Plum Tomatoes and Basil, page 49

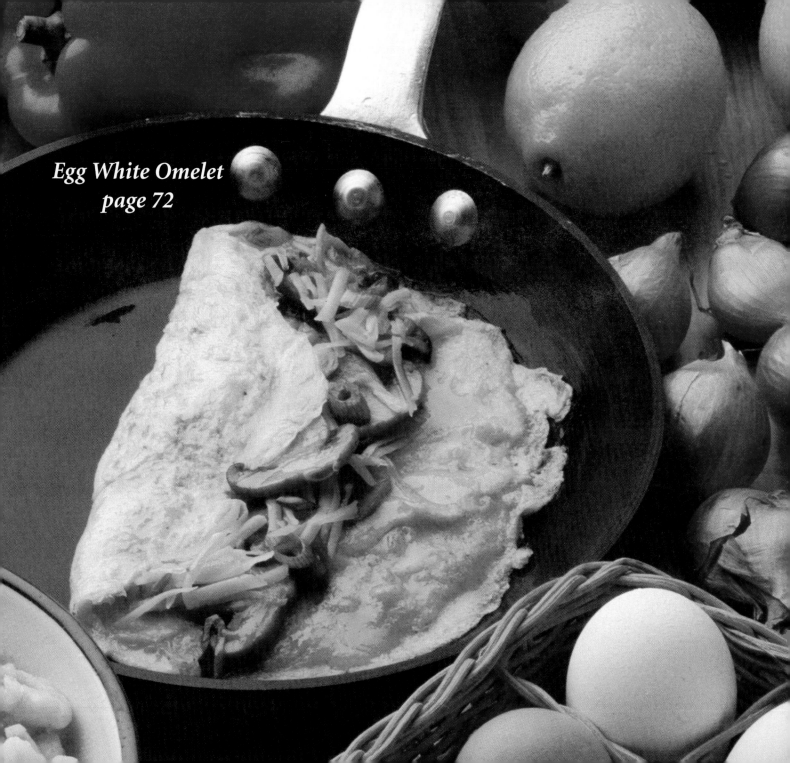

Egg White Omelet
page 72

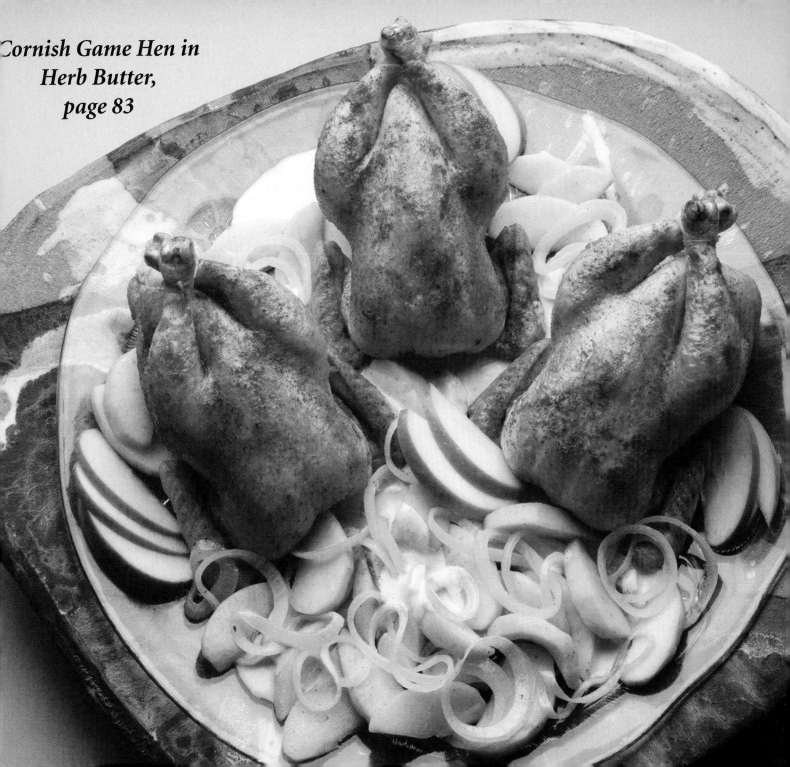

Cornish Game Hen in Herb Butter,
page 83

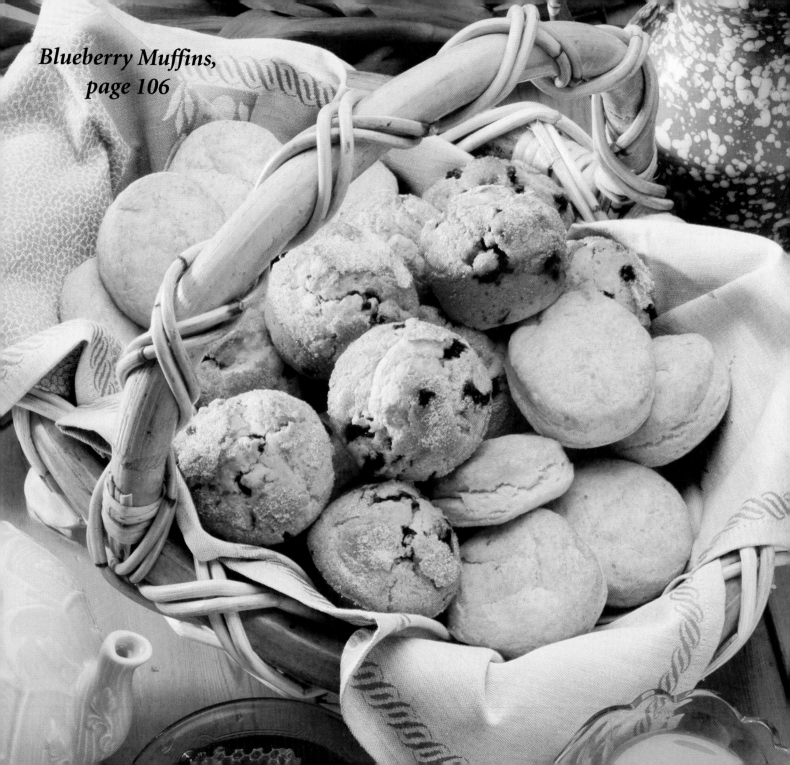

Blueberry Muffins,
page 106

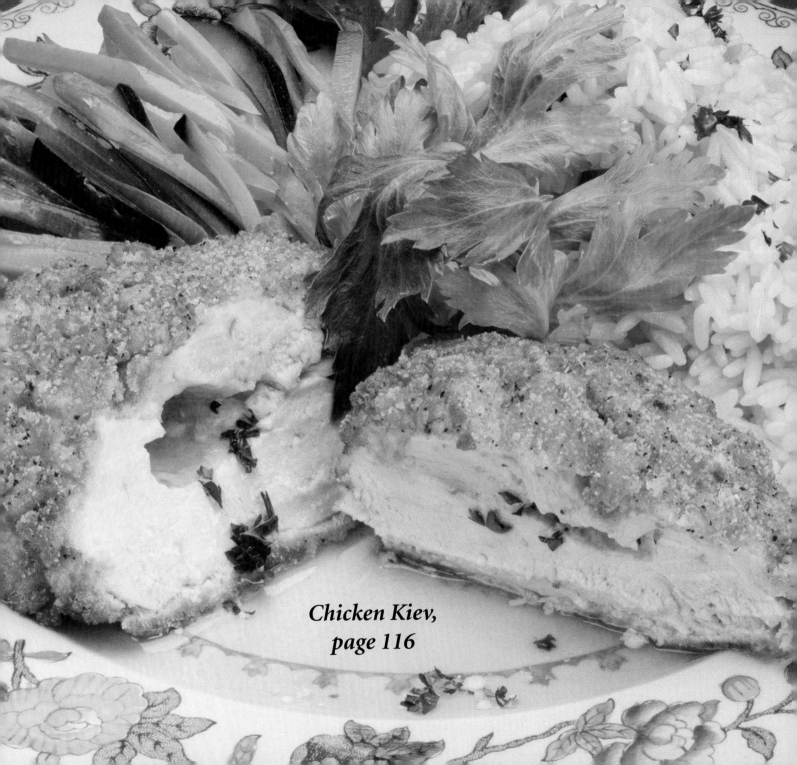

Chicken Kiev,
page 116

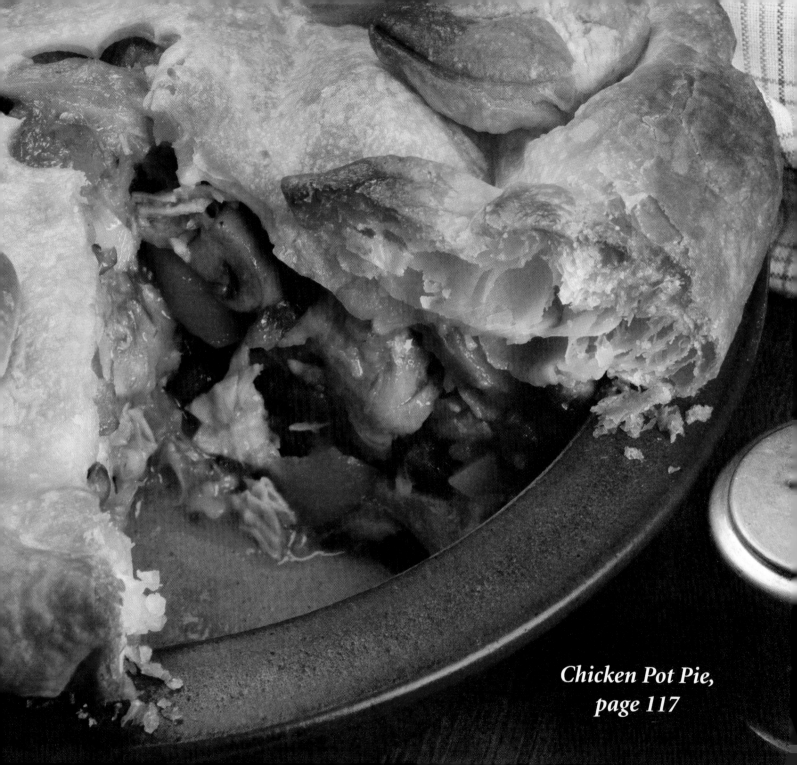

Chicken Pot Pie,
page 117

Mini-Meatballs with Spicy Marinara and Bow Tie Pasta

Ingredients

- 1 lb lean ground beef
- 1/4 lb ground turkey (97% fat free)
- 2 large eggs, beaten
- 3 Tbsp dry bread crumbs
- 1 medium onion, diced
- 2 Tbsp tomato paste
- 1 Tbsp Worcestershire sauce
- 2 tsp oregano
- 1 Tbsp fresh parsley, chopped
- 3 cups Spicy Marinara Sauce (see p. 148)
- 3 cups bow tie pasta, cooked

4 Servings
Serving Size: 1/2 cup pasta, 1 cup sauce

Calories	383
Calories from Fat	85
Total Fat	9 g
Saturated Fat	3 g
Cholesterol	85 mg
Sodium	258 mg
Carbohydrate	49 g
Dietary Fiber	4 g
Sugars	6 g
Protein	24 g

Exchanges
2 1/2 Starch
2 Lean Meat
1 1/2 Vegetable
1/2 Fat

Preparation

1. Preheat the oven to 350°F. Combine the beef, turkey, eggs, bread crumbs, onion, tomato paste, Worcestershire sauce, oregano, and parsley and gently mix. Using a tablespoon to measure, roll out the meat mixture into small balls. Place the meatballs on a baking sheet and bake for 15–20 minutes, or until the meatballs are done. Drain the extra grease from the baking sheet.
2. Serve the meatballs with Spicy Marinara Sauce overtop the bow tie pasta.

*P*ork Tenderloin Stuffed with Mushrooms and Leeks

Ingredients

- 2 pork tenderloins, about 1 1/4 lb total
- 1 Tbsp olive oil
- 1/2 lb mushrooms, sliced
- 1/2 leek, chopped
- 1/2 tsp salt
- 1/2 tsp pepper

---

4 Servings
Serving Size: 6.5 oz

Calories	308
Calories from Fat	110
Total Fat	12 g
Saturated Fat	3 g
Cholesterol	84 mg
Sodium	644 mg
Carbohydrate	16 g
Dietary Fiber	2 g
Sugars	>1 g
Protein	33 g

Exchanges
4 Very Lean Meat
1/2 Vegetable
2 Fat

Preparation

1. Preheat the oven to 350°F. Slice the tenderloins lengthwise, but only about three-quarters of the way through. Using a mallet or meat tenderizer, pound the tenderloin gently until it is level.
2. Heat the olive oil in a pan over medium heat. Add the mushrooms and cook for 2 minutes. Add the leeks and cook for 3–4 minutes, or until the leeks are tender. Remove the vegetables from the heat.
3. Season the tenderloins with salt and pepper. Place half the mushroom-leek mixture in the center of each tenderloin. Fold the tenderloin tightly so that there are no openings for the mixture to escape. Using butcher's twine, bind the tenderloin tightly so that it will not open during cooking.
4. Place the tenderloins in the oven and cook for 25–30 minutes, or until the internal temperature of each tenderloin is 155°F. Remove the tenderloins from the oven and let them rest for 3–5 minutes before cutting the twine and serving.

Chicken Cordon Bleu

Ingredients

- 2 boneless, skinless chicken breasts
- 4 slices lean ham
- 4 slices Swiss cheese
- 2 egg whites, slightly beaten
- 2 Tbsp low-fat (1%) milk
- 1 1/2 cups dry bread crumbs
- 1/2 Tbsp parsley
- 1 tsp garlic powder
- 1 tsp fresh oregano, chopped
- 1 tsp paprika
- 1 tsp fresh thyme, chopped
- 1/2 tsp black pepper

4 Servings

Serving Size: 1 chicken breast

Calories	308
Calories from Fat	107
Total Fat	12 g
Saturated Fat	7 g
Cholesterol	55 mg
Sodium	770 mg
Carbohydrate	24 g
Dietary Fiber	1 g
Sugars	1 g
Protein	25 g

Exchanges

1 1/2 Starch
2 Very Lean Meat
2 Fat

Preparation

1. Preheat the oven to 350°F. Using a mallet or meat tenderizer, pound the chicken breasts until they are 1/4-inch thick. Place 1 slice of ham and 1 slice of cheese on each breast. Roll the breasts and secure them with toothpicks to keep them from unrolling during cooking.
2. In a medium bowl, combine the egg whites and the milk. In a separate bowl, combine the bread crumbs and the remaining ingredients. Dredge the rolled chicken breasts through the egg mixture, then through the bread crumb mixture, until the chicken breasts are completely coated.
3. Spray a pan with nonstick cooking spray and heat over medium heat. Add the chicken breasts and brown all sides until golden brown. Remove the chicken breasts to a baking pan and place them in the oven. Cook for 15–20 minutes, or until chicken is done (internal temperature of 160°F). Remove from the oven and allow the chicken to rest for 5 minutes before serving.

Chicken Minute Steak Philly

Ingredients

- 4 boneless, skinless chicken breasts
- 1 tsp salt
- 1/2 tsp black pepper
- 2 Tbsp olive oil
- 1 green bell pepper, thinly sliced
- 1/2 medium onion, thinly sliced
- 4 hoagie rolls
- 4 slices low-fat mozzarella cheese

4 Servings
Serving Size: 1 hoagie

Calories	497
Calories from Fat	175
Total Fat	20 g
Saturated Fat	8 g
Cholesterol	88 mg
Sodium	1158 mg
Carbohydrate	37 g
Dietary Fiber	3 g
Sugars	4 g
Protein	42 g

Exchanges
2 Starch
4 1/2 Lean Meat
1/2 Vegetable
3 Fat

Preparation

1. Cut the chicken breasts into 3 long strips each. Season the chicken with salt and pepper. Heat 1 Tbsp of the olive oil in a pan over medium heat. Add the peppers and onion and cook until tender and slightly browned, about 5–7 minutes. Remove the peppers and onions and set aside.
2. Add the rest of the olive oil and the chicken. Cook the chicken 8–10 minutes, or until well done.
3. Slice the hoagie rolls lengthwise. Place the chicken, peppers, and onions inside. Add mozzarella cheese and serve immediately.

*B*aked Chicken Parmesan

Ingredients

1/2 cup dry bread crumbs
1/2 Tbsp oregano
  1 tsp basil
  1 tsp garlic powder
1/2 tsp black pepper
  1 large egg, beaten
1/4 cup low-fat (1%) milk
  4 boneless, skinless, chicken breasts
1/4 cup tomato sauce
  4 oz low-fat mozzarella cheese, grated
  2 oz Romano cheese, grated
  1 Tbsp fresh parsley, finely chopped

4 Servings
Serving Size: 1 chicken breast

Calories	359
Calories from Fat	123
Total Fat	14 g
Saturated Fat	7 g
Cholesterol	157 mg
Sodium	875 mg
Carbohydrate	13 g
Dietary Fiber	1 g
Sugars	2 g
Protein	43 g

Exchanges
1/2 Starch
3 1/2 Lean Meat
1 Fat

Preparation

1. Preheat the oven to 350°F. In a medium bowl, combine the bread crumbs, oregano, basil, garlic powder, and black pepper. In a separate bowl, combine the egg and milk. Dredge the chicken breasts through the egg mixture, then through the bread crumb mixture, until the chicken breasts are well coated. Bake the chicken breasts in the oven for 30–40 minutes, or until the chicken is done.
2. While the chicken is cooking, heat the tomato sauce and keep it in reserve. When the chicken is finished, cover each breast with sauce. Sprinkle the mozzarella and Romano cheeses overtop. Return the chicken to the oven for 5–7 minutes, or until the cheese is melted. Serve immediately and garnish with parsley.

Chicken Stir-fry

Ingredients

- 3 Tbsp sesame oil
- 4 boneless, skinless chicken breasts, cut into 1-inch strips
- 1 medium red bell pepper, julienned
- 1 medium yellow bell pepper, julienned
- 1 Tbsp garlic, minced
- 1 Tbsp fresh ginger, grated
- 1 small red onion, thinly sliced
- 1 cup broccoli florets
- 1/2 lb mushrooms, thinly sliced
- 2 Tbsp cornstarch
- 2 Tbsp water
- 2 Tbsp rice wine vinegar
- 4 Tbsp teriyaki sauce
- 3 Tbsp soy sauce
- 3 cups cooked white rice
- 4 green onions, chopped
- 1 Tbsp sesame seeds, toasted

4 Servings
Serving Size: 6 oz

Calories	343
Calories from Fat	124
Total Fat	14 g
Saturated Fat	3 g
Cholesterol	98 mg
Sodium	914 mg
Carbohydrate	14 g
Dietary Fiber	2 g
Sugars	3 g
Protein	40 g

Exchanges

4 1/2 Very Lean Meat
1 Vegetable
2 Fat

Preparation

1. Place the pan (or wok) on high heat. Add 1/2 of the sesame oil and 1/2 of the chicken and stir continuously. Cook for about 8–10 minutes, or until the chicken is thoroughly done. Remove the chicken from the pan, add the rest of your meat, and repeat. Set the cooked chicken aside on a separate plate.
2. Add the rest of the sesame oil. Add red and yellow bell peppers. Stir continuously for about 1 minute. Add the garlic, ginger, red onions, broccoli florets, and mushrooms. Continue to stir until the vegetables are tender, about 3–5 minutes.
3. In a small bowl, whisk together the cornstarch and water until it forms a smooth paste. Add the rice wine vinegar, teriyaki sauce, and the soy sauce to the pan. Slowly stir the cornstarch mixture into the pan and toss the ingredients to combine and thicken the sauce. Add the cooked chicken to the pan. Continue to toss all the ingredients until they are coated with the sauce.
4. Serve over 1/2 cup of cooked white rice and garnish with green onions and toasted sesame seeds.

Chef's Hints: Broccoli should be stored in the refrigerator in a plastic bag. After 3–5 days of storage, the flower of the broccoli begins to open and the vegetable loses some of its nutrients.

Herb-Crusted Chicken Breast

Ingredients

1/2 cup dry bread crumbs
1 1/2 tsp sage
1 tsp fresh rosemary, chopped
1 1/2 tsp fresh thyme, chopped
1/2 tsp black pepper
1/2 tsp garlic powder
1/2 tsp salt
1 large egg, beaten
4 boneless, skinless, chicken breasts

---

4 Servings
Serving Size: 1 chicken breast

Calories	212
Calories from Fat	42
Total Fat	5 g
Saturated Fat	1 g
Cholesterol	126 mg
Sodium	455 mg
Carbohydrate	10 g
Dietary Fiber	1 g
Sugars	1 g
Protein	30 g

Exchanges
1 Starch
1 Lean Meat
1 Fat

Preparation

1. Preheat the oven to 350°F. In a small bowl, combine the bread crumbs, sage, rosemary, thyme, black pepper, garlic powder, and salt. Dredge the chicken breasts through the beaten egg, then through the mixed herbs, until the chicken breasts are well coated. Place in the oven and cook for 20–30 minutes, or until the chicken is done (internal temperature of 160°F). Serve immediately.

*P*oached Chicken Breast Stuffed with Spinach and Swiss Cheese

Ingredients

4 boneless, skinless
  chicken breasts
  Pinch salt
  Pinch pepper
4 oz fresh or frozen
  spinach
4 slices Swiss cheese
6 cups water

4 Servings
Serving Size: 1 chicken
  breast

Calories	259
Calories from Fat	101
Total Fat	11 g
Saturated Fat	7 g
Cholesterol	98 mg
Sodium	162 mg
Carbohydrate	2 g
Dietary Fiber	1 g
Sugars	0 g
Protein	36 g

Exchanges
3 1/2 Very Lean Meat
1 Lean Meat
2 Fat

Preparation

1. Using a mallet or meat tenderizer, pound the chicken breasts until the meat is flat and even. Season the chicken with salt and pepper. Add a layer of spinach and a slice of Swiss cheese. Roll each breast tightly to ensure that the filling cannot escape. Wrap each breast tightly in plastic wrap. Water must not go inside.
2. In a deep pan, bring the water to a boil. Place the wrapped breasts into the water. Use a heat-proof plate to weigh the chicken breasts down and keep them completely submerged in the water. Allow them to simmer in the water for 20–25 minutes, or until the chicken is completely done. Remove the chicken from the water and let it cool for 5 minutes before serving.

*C*ornish Game Hen in Herb Butter

Ingredients

- 4 Cornish game hens (fresh or frozen: if frozen, allow to defrost fully in the refrigerator before beginning the recipe)
- 3/4 tsp salt
- 1/2 tsp white pepper
- 5 tsp olive oil
- 4 tsp Herb Butter (see p. 158)

4 Servings
Serving Size: 1/2 hen, skin removed

Calories	206
Calories from Fat	98
Total Fat	11 g
Saturated Fat	4 g
Cholesterol	127 mg
Sodium	288 mg
Carbohydrate	0 g
Dietary Fiber	0 g
Sugars	0 g
Protein	26 g

Exchanges
4 Lean Meat

4 Servings
Serving Size: 1/2 hen, including skin

Calories	393
Calories from Fat	270
Total Fat	30 g
Saturated Fat	9 g
Cholesterol	179 mg
Sodium	301 mg
Carbohydrate	0 g
Dietary Fiber	0 g
Sugars	0 g
Protein	29 g

Exchanges
4 Medium-Fat Meat
2 Fat

Preparation

1. Preheat the oven to 350°F. Discard the giblets and rinse out the inside of the hens. Season each hen by rubbing it with the salt and white pepper inside and out. Rub the olive oil onto the entire outer surface of each hen.
2. Place a large pan over medium-high heat. When the pan is fairly hot, place two of the hens in the pan, and sear them to a golden brown. Turn them over, and repeat on the other side. This will take about 30 seconds on each side. Repeat this process for the remaining 2 hens. (Note: Searing each hen is a necessary step in the cooking process, even though the high-fat skin is later discarded.)
3. Place the 4 hens on the rack of a roasting pan. Place the uncovered pan in the oven until the hens are fully cooked. (The hens are fully cooked when an instant-read thermometer, inserted in the breast, reads 170°F, or when the juices run clear when the hen is pierced with a fork.)
4. Remove the hens from the oven and allow them to cool for 5–7 minutes.
5. Using a sharp knife, carefully slice from the breast bone lengthwise down the breast, keeping the knife next to the bone. With the tip of the knife, follow through around the underside of the hen. Now, still using the tip of the knife, cut the breast away from the rest of the hen. Finally, cut the leg and thigh piece away. Remove the skins and arrange 1 breast and 1 leg-and-thigh piece (1/2 hen) on each plate. Melt 1 tsp of the Herb Butter on each portion and serve.

Chef's Hints: Note how much more fat is added when the skin is left on the hen in this recipe. People who are looking to cut their fat intake—and we all should be trying—are advised to remove the skin before eating.

Roasted Turkey

Ingredients

1 10–12 lb whole turkey
1 tsp salt
2 tsp black pepper
1 Tbsp garlic, minced
3 sprigs fresh rosemary
7–8 sprigs fresh thyme
3 sprigs fresh oregano
2 Tbsp olive oil

16 Servings
Serving Size: 4.5 oz

Calories	288
Calories from Fat	138
Total Fat	16 g
Saturated Fat	4 g
Cholesterol	97 mg
Sodium	225 mg
Carbohydrate	1 g
Dietary Fiber	0 g
Sugars	0 g
Protein	35 g

Exchanges
5 Lean Meat
1/2 Fat

Preparation

1. Preheat the oven to 400°F. Remove the turkey from its wrapping, and remove all the items from its internal cavity. Rinse the inside with water and pat dry with a paper towel. Season the cavity with the salt, pepper, and garlic by rubbing these items into the internal wall of the cavity. Add the rosemary, thyme, and oregano to the internal cavity. Rub the olive oil over the outer skin of the turkey.

2. Place the turkey in a roasting pan in the oven. After 15 minutes, lower the oven temperature to 325°F. Continue to cook until the turkey reaches an internal temperature of 165°F, about 2–2 1/2 hours. When the turkey is done, let it rest for 10 minutes before serving.

Flavor Idea: Try this flavorful turkey for your next Thanksgiving dinner. The fresh herbs give the meat a great taste and fill the house with a wonderful smell. Serve it with Easy Stuffing (see p. 159).

Turkey Sausage with Spinach and Bow Tie Pasta

Ingredients

  2 quarts water
1/2 lb bow tie pasta
1/2 lb ground turkey (97% fat free)
1/2 Tbsp garlic, minced
1/4 Tbsp caraway seeds
1/2 Tbsp sage
1/2 Tbsp fresh rosemary, finely chopped
     Nonstick cooking spray
  1 pint Chicken Stock (see p. 155)
  8 oz fresh or frozen spinach
  1 Tbsp butter
     Pinch black pepper

---

5 Servings

Serving Size: 3/4 cup pasta, 1/2 cup turkey and spinach mixture.

Calories	287
Calories from Fat	92
Total Fat	10 g
Saturated Fat	4 g
Cholesterol	70 mg
Sodium	121 mg
Carbohydrate	29 g
Dietary Fiber	2 g
Sugars	1 g
Protein	20 g

Exchanges

2 Starch
2 Lean Meat
1 Fat

Preparation

1. In a medium pot, bring the water to a boil. Add the bow tie pasta and cook for 8–12 minutes, or until the pasta is done.
2. Combine the ground turkey, garlic, caraway seeds, sage, and rosemary in a medium bowl. Mix gently. Spray a pan with nonstick cooking spray and heat over medium heat. Add the turkey mixture and cook, stirring to break up the meat, until it is almost done, about 3–4 minutes. Add the chicken stock and bring the liquid to a simmer. Allow the liquid to reduce by half, then remove the ground turkey and set aside.
3. Clean the spinach under cold, running water. Remove the stems and pat the spinach dry. Chop the spinach roughly. Heat the butter in a pan over medium heat. Add the spinach and stir quickly until it wilts, about 1 minute. Season with black pepper.
4. Serve the turkey sausage and spinach over the bow tie pasta. Drizzle 1 Tbsp of the chicken stock over the noodles.

Broiled Lamb Chops with Onion Confit

Ingredients

2 tsp olive oil
1 lb red onion, sliced
4 Tbsp balsamic vinegar
1 Tbsp orange rind, grated
4 1-inch thick lamb chops,
   about 5–6 oz each
   black pepper, to taste

---

4 Servings
Serving Size: 1 chop

Calories	281
Calories from Fat	156
Total Fat	17 g
Saturated Fat	7 g
Cholesterol	64 mg
Sodium	57 mg
Carbohydrate	14 g
Dietary Fiber	3 g
Sugars	9 g
Protein	18 g

Exchanges
2 1/2 Lean Meat
2 Vegetable
2 Fat

Preparation

1. Heat the olive oil in a large pan over medium heat. Add the red onions. Do not stir. Let the onions turn light brown, then turn and brown on the other side. When the onions are almost done, add the balsamic vinegar and orange rind. Cook for 2–3 minutes, until the liquid is almost gone. Remove the onion confit and set aside.

2. Preheat the oven broiler. Season the lamb chops with black pepper and olive oil and place on a roasting rack in the oven. Cook 12–16 minutes, or until the lamb is done. Serve lamb chops topped with onion confit immediately.

Baked Catfish Nuggets

Ingredients

1 lb catfish, cut into 3/4-inch nuggets
1/2 tsp black pepper
1 tsp garlic powder
4 large eggs, beaten
1/2 cup all-purpose flour
Nonstick cooking spray

4 Servings
Serving Size: 1/4 of the recipe

Calories	264
Calories from Fat	65
Total Fat	7 g
Saturated Fat	2 g
Cholesterol	241 mg
Sodium	105 mg
Carbohydrate	19 g
Dietary Fiber	1 g
Sugars	1 g
Protein	28 g

Exchanges
1 Starch
3 1/2 Very Lean Meat
1 Lean Meat
1 Fat

Preparation

1. Preheat the oven to 375°F. Toss the catfish nuggets with the black pepper and garlic powder. Dip the nuggets in the beaten egg, then dredge the nuggets in the flour until they are well coated.
2. Spray a baking sheet with nonstick cooking spray. Arrange the nuggets on the baking sheet and place them in the oven. Cook for 20–25 minutes, or until the catfish nuggets are done.

Baked Salmon Fish Sticks

Ingredients

1 cup yellow corn meal
1 tsp black pepper
1 tsp garlic powder
1 lb salmon, skinless and
   cut into 2-inch slices
1 cup low-fat (1%) milk
   Nonstick cooking spray

4 Servings
Serving Size: 1/4 recipe

Calories	207
Calories from Fat	50
Total Fat	6 g
Saturated Fat	1 g
Cholesterol	77 mg
Sodium	108 mg
Carbohydrate	8 g
Dietary Fiber	1 g
Sugars	1 g
Protein	30 g

Exchanges
1/2 Starch
4 1/2 Very Lean Meat
1/2 Fat

Preparation

1. Preheat the oven to 375°F. Combine the corn meal, black pepper, and garlic powder. Dip the salmon pieces in the milk, then dredge them in the corn meal mixture until thoroughly coated.
2. Spray a baking sheet with nonstick cooking spray, then arrange the salmon sticks on it. Bake in the oven for 25–30 minutes, or until the sticks break apart with ease.

Poached Salmon with Dill, Cinnamon, and Honeydew Salsa

Ingredients

2 cups medium honey-
dew melon, diced

1/4 cup red onion, diced

1/4 cup red bell pepper,
diced

1 Tbsp jalapeño pepper,
minced

1 Tbsp honey

1 Tbsp fresh cilantro,
chopped

4 salmon filets, about
4-oz each

4 sprigs fresh dill

2 tsp cinnamon

1 tsp black pepper

2 quarts water

4 Servings
Serving Size: 1 filet,
3/4 cup salsa

Calories	392
Calories from Fat	155
Total Fat	17 g
Saturated Fat	3 g
Cholesterol	135 mg
Sodium	112 mg
Carbohydrate	15 g
Dietary Fiber	2 g
Sugars	12 g
Protein	43 g

Exchanges

1/2 Starch

6 Lean Meat

1/2 Fruit

Preparation

1. Combine the honeydew, red onion, red bell pepper, jalapeño, honey, and cilantro together. Cover and refrigerate.
2. Lay out a 10-inch sheet of plastic wrap. Place a piece of salmon in the center of the plastic wrap. Place 1 sprig of dill, 1/2 tsp of cinnamon, and 1/4 tsp of black pepper on top of salmon. Fold the plastic wrap over the salmon and wrap it tightly on all ends. Repeat the process for the other salmon filets.
3. In a medium pot, bring the water to a boil. Place the four pieces of wrapped salmon in the water. Cook for 20 minutes, or until the salmon is done. Serve immediately with honeydew salsa.

Shrimp and Scallop Stew

Ingredients

1/2 lb potatoes, diced
1/2 cup carrots, diced
  2 Tbsp olive oil
1/2 cup onion, diced
1/2 Tbsp garlic, minced
1/4 lb mushrooms, sliced
  4 oz shrimp, deveined
     and without shells
  4 oz bay scallops
1/4 cup white wine
  1 cup evaporated skim
     milk
  2 Tbsp cornstarch
  2 Tbsp water
1/2 cup green onions,
     chopped
1/2 Tbsp fresh dill,
     chopped
1/2 tsp salt
     Pinch black pepper

5 Servings
Serving Size: 1 cup.

Calories	185
Calories from Fat	36
Total Fat	4 g
Saturated Fat	1 g
Cholesterol	53 mg
Sodium	449 mg
Carbohydrate	22 g
Dietary Fiber	2 g
Sugars	9 g
Protein	14 g

Exchanges

1/2 Starch
1 Very Lean Meat
1 Vegetable
1 Fat

Preparation

1. Fill a medium pot with water and bring it to a boil. Add the potatoes. Cook for 5 minutes. Add the diced carrots. Cook for 5 minutes more, or until the vegetables are tender. Remove the vegetables from the water and set aside.
2. Heat 1 Tbsp of the olive oil in a large pot over medium heat. Add the onion and garlic and cook until translucent, about 5 minutes. Add the mushrooms and cook until they are slightly wilted, about 3–5 minutes. Remove them from the pot and set aside.
3. Add the remaining 1 Tbsp of olive oil to the pot, then add the shrimp and scallops. Cook for 2–3 minutes. Add the white wine and allow it to reduce by half. Add all of the cooked vegetables to the pot, plus the evaporated milk. Bring the liquid to a simmer. In a separate bowl, mix the cornstarch and water until they form a smooth paste. Slowly stir the cornstarch mixture into the pan to thicken the liquid. Return the liquid to a simmer, then remove it from the heat.
4. Add the green onions and dill. Season with salt and pepper. Serve immediately.

Stuffed Flounder over Linguine with Spicy Roasted Red Pepper Puree

Ingredients

10 red bell peppers
1 tsp olive oil
1 Tbsp garlic, minced
1 jalapeño pepper, finely chopped
1 cup white wine
1 cup Chicken Stock (see p. 155)
1 tsp black pepper
4 flounder filets, skinless and boneless
8 oz lump crab meat
2 tsp black pepper
2 Tbsp lemon juice
2 tsp butter, melted
3 quarts water
1 lb linguini pasta
2 tsp salt

4 Servings

Serving Size: 1 filet, 1/2 cup pasta

Calories	397
Calories from Fat	38
Total Fat	4 g
Saturated Fat	1 g
Cholesterol	66 mg
Sodium	173 mg
Carbohydrate	56 g
Dietary Fiber	6 g
Sugars	6 g
Protein	30 g

Exchanges

3 Starch
3 Very Lean Meat
2 Vegetables
1/2 Fat

Preparation

1. Place the red bell peppers directly on the burners of a gas stove and turn the heat on high. Allow the skin to turn completely black, turning the pepper occasionally. When all the peppers are blackened, put them in a large bowl and cover with plastic wrap to steam the skins. After 10 minutes, run the peppers under cold water and peel away the skins. Remove the tops and seeds of the peppers; roughly chop the rest.
2. Heat 1 tsp of the olive oil in a medium pot over medium heat. Add the garlic and jalapeño and cook for about 1 minute until the garlic turns white. Add the chopped red peppers, white wine, and chicken stock. Bring the liquid to a simmer for 30 minutes, or until the red peppers are very tender. Strain the liquid into a small bowl and keep it.
3. Place the red pepper mixture into a food processor and puree. If the sauce is too thick, add some of the strained liquid. Season the sauce with black pepper and set it aside.
4. Preheat the oven to 350°F. With a sharp knife, make a 3-inch cut down the length of the flounder filet without cutting through it. Turn the knife so it is almost parallel to the cutting board and make another slice to create a pocket on one side of the filet. Repeat the process on the other side. Place 2 Tbsp of the crab meat into the pocket of the flounder. Place the flounder on a baking dish and season with black pepper, lemon juice, and butter. Bake for 20 minutes, or until the filet is white and flaky.
5. While the flounder is baking, bring the water to a boil. Add the salt and pasta and stir immediately to prevent the pasta sticking. Cook the pasta for 8–10 minutes, or until done. Drain the pasta.
6. Toss the pasta with the red pepper sauce and serve the flounder filet on top of the pasta.

Chef's Hints: This recipe looks hard, but it is worth the effort. Not only do the roasted peppers make it intensely flavorful, but it is also very low in fat.

Crab Ravioli with Spinach Sauce

Ingredients

- 8 oz lump crab meat
- Pinch white pepper
- 1 tsp lemon juice
- 1 egg, beaten
- 1/4 cup water
- 1 12-oz package won ton wrappers
- 1 tsp olive oil
- 1 small onion, minced
- 1 10-oz package frozen spinach
- 1/2 cup Chicken Stock (see p. 155)
- Pinch salt
- Pinch white pepper

4 Servings
Serving Size: about 6–7 ravioli, 1/2 cup sauce

Calories	312
Calories from Fat	18
Total Fat	2 g
Saturated Fat	>1 g
Cholesterol	47 mg
Sodium	690 mg
Carbohydrate	51 g
Dietary Fiber	3 g
Sugars	2 g
Protein	21 g

Exchanges

3 Starch
1 1/2 Very Lean Meat
1 Vegetable

Preparation

1. Combine the crab meat, white pepper, and lemon juice. In a separate bowl, mix the egg and water. Brush a won ton wrapper with the egg mixture, place 1 tsp of the crab mixture in the center, and lay another won ton wrapper over the first. Squeeze the air out of the center of the wrappers as you seal the edges together. Place the finished wrappers under a moist towel to prevent them from drying out. Repeat until all the crab mixture has been used.

2. Heat the olive oil in a pan over medium heat. Add the onions and cook until translucent, about 5 minutes. Add the spinach and cook until it is wilted. Add the chicken stock, salt, and white pepper. Bring the liquid to a simmer for 5 minutes. Pour the spinach mixture into a food processor and puree until smooth.

3. In a large pot, bring water and 1 tsp of salt to a boil. Add the ravioli and cook for 3–5 minutes. Remove the ravioli from the water and serve with the spinach sauce immediately.

Lentil Soup

Ingredients

- 1 tsp olive oil
- 2/3 medium onion, finely diced
- 2/3 medium carrot, finely diced
- 1/3 stalk celery, finely diced
- 1 tsp garlic, minced
- 1 quart Chicken Stock (see p. 155)
- 1/3 lb lentils
- 1/3 tsp fresh thyme, minced
- 4 tsp balsamic vinegar
- 1 Tbsp fresh parsley leaves, chopped

6 Servings
Serving Size: about 1 cup.

Calories	101
Calories from Fat	15
Total Fat	2 g
Saturated Fat	1 g
Cholesterol	2 mg
Sodium	159 mg
Carbohydrate	16 g
Dietary Fiber	6 g
Sugars	3 g
Protein	7 g

Exchanges
1 Starch
1/2 Vegetable
1/2 Fat

Preparation

1. Heat the olive oil in a large pot over medium heat. Add the onion, carrot, and celery. Cook until the vegetables are slightly tender, about 3–4 minutes. Add the garlic and cook for 1 minute. Add the chicken stock, lentils, and thyme. Bring the liquid to a simmer. Cover and cook for 1 hour, or until the lentils are tender but still whole. Add the balsamic vinegar. Serve with parsley as a garnish.

Chef's Hints: When choosing celery look for solid stalks. Do not purchase celery if even one stalk is wilted. Celery only stores in the refrigerator for 7–10 days.

Minestrone Soup

Ingredients

1/2 Tbsp olive oil
1/2 medium onion, finely diced
1/4 medium carrot, finely diced
1/4 stalk celery, finely diced
2/3 tsp garlic, minced
2 Tbsp leeks, finely diced
3 oz (about 1/3 cup) canned tomatoes, chopped
1/2 medium zucchini, diced
1/4 tsp fresh thyme, minced
3/4 tsp fresh oregano, minced
3 cups Chicken Stock (see p. 155)
3 oz (about 1/2 cup) frozen spinach, chopped
3/4 cup white beans, cooked
1/4 tsp salt
1/8 tsp white pepper
1 tsp Parmesan cheese, grated

4 Servings

Serving Size: about 1 cup

Calories	110
Calories from Fat	29
Total Fat	3 g
Saturated Fat	1 g
Cholesterol	3 mg
Sodium	283 mg
Carbohydrate	15 g
Dietary Fiber	5 g
Sugars	3 g
Protein	7 g

Exchanges

1 Starch
1/2 Lean Meat
1 Vegetable
1/2 Fat

Preparation

1. Heat the olive oil in a medium pot over medium heat. Add the onion, carrot, and celery. Cook until the vegetables are slightly tender, about 3–4 minutes. Add the garlic and leek and cook for 1 minute. Add the tomato, zucchini, thyme, oregano, and chicken stock. Bring the liquid to a simmer for 20 minutes.

2. Add the spinach and white beans. Return the liquid to a simmer for 20 minutes. Season with the salt and white pepper. Serve immediately and garnish with the Parmesan cheese.

*T*omato and Mozzarella Salad

Ingredients

- 2 cups balsamic vinegar
- 2 large tomatoes
- 8 oz low-fat mozzarella
- 1 small red onion, diced small
- 2 Tbsp extra virgin olive oil
- 10 leaves fresh basil, cut into thin strips
     fresh black pepper

4 Servings
Serving Size: 1/4 of salad

Calories	303
Calories from Fat	147
Total Fat	16 g
Saturated Fat	6 g
Cholesterol	27 mg
Sodium	421 mg
Carbohydrate	24 g
Dietary Fiber	1 g
Sugars	20 g
Protein	18 g

Exchanges
1 Other Carbohydrate
2 Lean Meat
1 Vegetable
2 Fat

Preparation

1. Place the balsamic vinegar in a small pot over medium-high heat. Allow the liquid to reduce by half, then set it aside to cool.
2. Slice the tomatoes into medium-thick slices and arrange them on a plate. Slice the cheese in medium slices and arrange cheese slices between the slices of tomato. Sprinkle the red onions overtop. Pour the oil, then the balsamic vinegar, overtop the dish. Garnish the plate with the basil and pepper and serve.

Cajun Baked Sweet Potato

Ingredients

1/2 Tbsp paprika
1 tsp brown sugar
1/4 tsp black pepper
1/4 tsp onion powder
1/4 tsp thyme
1/4 tsp rosemary
1/4 tsp garlic powder
1/8 tsp cayenne pepper
2 large sweet potatoes
1/2 Tbsp olive oil

4 Servings
Serving Size: 1/2 potato

Calories	81
Calories from Fat	12
Total Fat	1 g
Saturated Fat	0 g
Cholesterol	0 mg
Sodium	9 mg
Carbohydrate	16 g
Dietary Fiber	2 g
Sugars	4 g
Protein	1 g

Exchanges
1 Starch

Preparation

1. Preheat the oven to 375°F. Combine the paprika, brown sugar, black pepper, onion powder, thyme, rosemary, garlic powder, and cayenne pepper. Slice the sweet potatoes in half lengthwise. Rub the halves with oil, then rub the seasoning mix over the open half of each potato. Bake for 1 hour, or until the sweet potatoes are tender.

Paprika Potatoes

Ingredients

3/4 lb red potatoes, cut into quarters
2 Tbsp unsalted butter, melted
1 Tbsp paprika
1/2 tsp black pepper
1/2 tsp salt

4 Servings
Serving Size: about 3/4 cup

Calories	187
Calories from Fat	108
Total Fat	12 g
Saturated Fat	7 g
Cholesterol	31 mg
Sodium	588 mg
Carbohydrate	19 g
Dietary Fiber	2 g
Sugars	1 g
Protein	2 g

Exchanges
1 Starch
2 Fat

Preparation

1. Preheat the oven to 350°F. Pour the melted butter over the potatoes. Add the paprika, black pepper, and salt. Mix well so that the potatoes are evenly coated. Bake in the oven for 30–35 minutes, or until the potatoes are fully cooked.

Whipped Sweet Potatoes with Caramelized Shallots

Ingredients

- 1 tsp olive oil
- 3 oz shallots, cut into 1/4-inch pieces
- 2 quarts water
- 1 lb fresh sweet potatoes, peeled and diced into 1-inch pieces
- 1 tsp salt
- 1/4 cup evaporated skim milk
- 2 Tbsp margarine
- 1/4 tsp white pepper
- 1/4 tsp cinnamon or nutmeg

8 Servings
Serving Size: 1/8 recipe.

Calories	93
Calories from Fat	31
Total Fat	3 g
Saturated Fat	1 g
Cholesterol	0 mg
Sodium	53 mg
Carbohydrate	14 g
Dietary Fiber	2 g
Sugars	6 g
Protein	2 g

Exchanges
1 Starch
1/2 Fat

Preparation

1. Heat the olive oil in a pan over medium-high heat. Add the shallots and cook until they turn golden, about 3–5 minutes. Remove from the pan and set aside.
2. In a medium pot, bring the water to a boil. Add the sweet potatoes and the salt. Return the water to a boil and cook for 10–15 minutes, or until the potatoes are tender. Drain the water.
3. Using an electric hand mixer, combine the sweet potatoes, half of the cooked shallots, and the remaining ingredients until they are thoroughly mixed. Serve immediately with the remaining shallots as a garnish.

Roasted Baby Carrots

Ingredients

1 1/2 cup orange juice
1 lb baby carrots
1 Tbsp olive oil
1/4 tsp salt
1/8 tsp white pepper

---

4 Servings
Serving Size: about 1/2 cup

Calories	112
Calories from Fat	38
Total Fat	4 g
Saturated Fat	1 g
Cholesterol	0 mg
Sodium	622 mg
Carbohydrate	18 g
Dietary Fiber	2 g
Sugars	14 g
Protein	2 g

Exchanges
1/2 Fruit
2 Vegetable
1 Fat

Preparation

1. Preheat the oven to 400°F. Bring the orange juice to a boil in a pan, then reduce the heat to a simmer. Allow the liquid to reduce by one-fourth. Remove from the heat and allow it to cool.
2. Combine the remaining ingredients in a baking dish and mix well. Bake for 20 minutes, then stir the carrots to brown the other side. Bake for another 20 minutes. Serve with the reduced orange juice as a sauce.

Did You Know? The best way to reduce produce spoilage is to let air circulate in the storage bags. Next time you seal your vegetables shut, keep the bags filled with air.

Spaghetti Squash Casserole

Ingredients

1 medium spaghetti squash
1 cup cold water
2 cups low-fat Swiss cheese (or Gruyere), grated
1 Tbsp Three Pepper Butter (see p. 153)

4 Servings
Serving Size: about 1/2 cup.

Calories	129
Calories from Fat	48
Total Fat	5 g
Saturated Fat	3 g
Cholesterol	23 mg
Sodium	129 mg
Carbohydrate	8 g
Dietary Fiber	1 g
Sugars	1 g
Protein	13 g

Exchanges
2 Very Lean Meat
1 Vegetable
1 Fat

Preparation

1. Preheat the oven to 350°F. Cut the squash in half lengthwise. Using a spoon, remove the seeds and discard. Place the squash in a large baking dish open side down and cover with the water. Bake for 30 minutes, or until the squash is tender. Remove from the oven and allow it to cool.
2. Scrape the meat of the squash away from the rind using a fork. Combine the squash meat in a baking dish with the Swiss cheese and the butter. Bake in the oven for 20 minutes. Serve immediately.

Steamed Cauliflower with Dill

Ingredients

- 3 cups water
- 1 head cauliflower, leaves removed
- 2 Tbsp fresh dill, chopped
- 1/4 tsp white pepper
- 1 lemon

4 Servings
Serving Size: 1/4 recipe

Calories	38
Calories from Fat	0
Total Fat	0 g
Saturated Fat	0 g
Cholesterol	0 mg
Sodium	44 mg
Carbohydrate	8 g
Dietary Fiber	3 g
Sugars	3 g
Protein	3 g

Exchanges
1 1/2 Vegetable

Preparation

1. Bring the water to a boil in a large pot. Add the cauliflower, dill, and white pepper. Cover and steam for 20 minutes. Serve with lemon juice squeezed overtop.

Vegetable Stir-fry

Ingredients

2 tsp sesame oil
1 tsp fresh ginger, minced
1 Tbsp garlic, minced
2 medium carrots, cut into matchsticks
1/4 lb white mushrooms, quartered
2 tsp hot bean paste
2 tsp water
1 medium red bell pepper, thinly sliced
1 medium yellow bell pepper, thinly sliced
1 medium green bell pepper, thinly sliced
3/4 cup zucchini, sliced
2 green onions, chopped

4 Servings
Serving Size: about 1 cup

Calories	89
Calories from Fat	24
Total Fat	3 g
Saturated Fat	0 g
Cholesterol	0 mg
Sodium	31 mg
Carbohydrate	16 g
Dietary Fiber	4 g
Sugars	5 g
Protein	3 g

Exchanges
2 Vegetable
1/2 Fat

Preparation

1. In a large pan or wok, heat the oil over medium-high heat. Add the ginger and garlic and stir for 30 seconds. Add the carrots and mushrooms and stir for 2 minutes. Combine the bean paste and water until it is smooth and add it to the pan. Add the remaining ingredients and stir continuously for about 2–3 minutes, or until all the vegetables are tender.

Orange and Polenta Soufflé

Ingredients

- 1 Tbsp butter
- 6 Tbsp sugar
- 6 medium oranges
- 8 oz evaporated skim milk
- 1/2 cup corn meal
- 3/4 cup egg whites

4 Servings
Serving Size: 1 soufflé

Calories	380
Calories from Fat	114
Total Fat	13 g
Saturated Fat	7 g
Cholesterol	33 mg
Sodium	158 mg
Carbohydrate	59 g
Dietary Fiber	3 g
Sugars	31 g
Protein	11 g

Exchanges
2 1/2 Other Carbohydrate
1/2 Very Lean Meat
1/2 Fruit
2 1/2 Fat

Preparation

1. Preheat the oven to 400°F. Lightly coat the soufflé molds with butter, then dust each with 1 Tbsp of sugar.
2. Juice the oranges into a small pot. Reduce the liquid by three-quarters over medium-high heat. Add the evaporated skim milk and return the liquid to a simmer. Immediately remove from the heat and allow it to steep for 30 minutes.
3. Strain the liquid into a new pot and bring it to a simmer. Add 1 Tbsp of sugar, then add the corn meal in a slow stream while stirring constantly. Bring the pot to a simmer and continue to stir until the mixture pulls away from the sides of the pot. Remove from the heat and set aside.
4. Beat the egg whites until it forms a heavy foam, then gradually beat in 1 Tbsp of sugar. Continue to beat the egg whites until medium peaks form. Fold the egg whites into the corn meal mixture. Pour the mix into the prepared molds.
5. Place the molds in a roasting pan, then fill the pan with water until the level is half the height of the molds. Bake for 18–20 minutes, or until the soufflés have risen and are golden and creamy in the center.

Did You Know? There are two different kinds of corn meal: steel ground and stone (or water) ground. Steel ground corn meal is processed once most of the husk and germ is removed. Stone (or water) ground corn meal retains a large portion of the germ.

Crepes Stuffed with Bosc Pears Poached in Cabernet Sauvignon

Ingredients

1 cup all-purpose flour
Pinch salt
1 cup egg whites
1 cup reduced-fat (2%) milk
Nonstick cooking spray
2 quarts water
2 Bosc pears
3 cups Cabernet Sauvignon red wine
1 Tbsp orange rind, grated
1/2 cup orange juice
1 tsp lemon rind, grated
1 Tbsp honey

---

4 Servings
Serving Size: 2 crepes

Calories	130
Calories from Fat	5
Total Fat	>1 g
Saturated Fat	0 g
Cholesterol	1 mg
Sodium	25 mg
Carbohydrate	19 g
Dietary Fiber	2 g
Sugars	11 g
Protein	2 g

Exchanges
1/2 Starch
1 Fruit

Preparation

1. Sift the flour and add a pinch salt. In a separate bowl, combine the egg whites and the milk. Slowly whisk the dry and wet ingredients together until they are smooth. Spray a small, nonstick pan with nonstick cooking spray and heat it over medium-high heat. Coat the bottom of the pan with a small amount of the crepe mixture and let it cook. When it is lightly golden on one side, flip the crepe and cook the other side until lightly golden. Repeat until the crepe mixture is gone.

2. Bring the 2 quarts of water to a boil and add the pears. Keep the pears submerged in boiling water for 2 minutes, then remove them to a bowl of ice water. Let the pears cool for 3–4 minutes, then use a paring knife to remove the skin from each pear. Slice each pear in half and cut away the core.

3. In a medium pot, combine the remaining ingredients and bring to a simmer. Add the halved pears and cook for 15 minutes, or until the pears are tender. Remove the pears, then continue to simmer the liquid until it has been reduced by three-quarters. Remove from the heat and set aside.

4. Preheat the oven to 350°F. Slice the pears thinly. Place 6–7 of the slices in the center of each crepe. Roll the crepes and place them in a baking dish. Bake for 15 minutes. Serve each crepe with 2 Tbsp of the wine sauce.

*E*asy Muffins

Ingredients

- 2/3 cup sugar
- 1/2 tsp salt
- 2 1/2 cups all-purpose flour
- 1 Tbsp baking powder
- 1 large egg
- 1/3 cup vegetable oil
- 1 1/4 cups reduced-fat (2%) milk
- 1 tsp vanilla extract

12 Servings
Serving Size: 1 muffin

Calories	206
Calories from Fat	63
Total Fat	7 g
Saturated Fat	1 g
Cholesterol	19 mg
Sodium	191 mg
Carbohydrate	32 g
Dietary Fiber	1 g
Sugars	12 g
Protein	4 g

Exchanges
2 Starch
1 1/2 Fat

Preparation

1. Preheat the oven to 400°F. Combine the sugar, salt, flour, and baking powder. In a separate bowl, combine the liquid ingredients. Make a well in the center of the dry ingredients and add the liquid ingredients. Mix with a fork until it forms a loose batter.
2. Lightly coat a muffin pan with nonstick cooking spray. Spoon the batter into the pan until the cups are 3/4 filled. Bake for 18–20 minutes, or until the tops are golden brown and the centers are firm.

*E*asy Blueberry Muffins

Ingredients

2/3 cup sugar
1/2 tsp salt
2 1/2 cups all-purpose flour
1 Tbsp baking powder
1 large egg
1/3 cup vegetable oil
1 1/4 cups reduced-fat (2%) milk
1 tsp vanilla extract
1 cup fresh or frozen blueberries

12 Servings
Serving Size: 1 muffin

Calories	227
Calories from Fat	65
Total Fat	7 g
Saturated Fat	1 g
Cholesterol	19 mg
Sodium	193 mg
Carbohydrate	37 g
Dietary Fiber	2 g
Sugars	16 g
Protein	4 g

Exchanges
2 Starch
1/2 Fruit
1 1/2 Fat

Preparation

3. Preheat the oven to 400°F. Combine the sugar, salt, flour, and baking powder. In a separate bowl, combine the liquid ingredients. Make a well in the center of the dry ingredients and add the liquid ingredients and the blueberries. Mix with a fork until it forms a loose batter.

4. Lightly coat a muffin pan with nonstick cooking spray. Spoon the batter into the pan until the cups are 3/4 filled. Bake for 18–20 minutes, or until the tops are golden brown and the centers are firm.

Did You Know? New Jersey is the largest producer of blueberries, followed by Michigan.

Pumpkin Parfait with Berries and Low-Fat Whipped Topping

Ingredients

1 1/2 cups pumpkin puree (not pumpkin pie mix)
1 Tbsp sugar
1/8 tsp nutmeg
1/8 tsp ground cloves
1/2 cup evaporated skim milk
10 Tbsp low-fat whipped topping
1 cup fresh or frozen raspberries
1/2 tsp cinnamon

4 Servings
Serving Size: 1 parfait

Calories	108
Calories from Fat	16
Total Fat	2 g
Saturated Fat	1 g
Cholesterol	1 mg
Sodium	44 mg
Carbohydrate	20 g
Dietary Fiber	5 g
Sugars	12 g
Protein	4 g

Exchanges
1 1/2 Other Carbohydrate

Preparation

1. Combine the pumpkin puree with the sugar, nutmeg, and cloves. Slowly fold in the evaporated skim milk and 2 Tbsp of the whipped topping. Cover and refrigerate until ready to serve.
2. When ready to serve, spoon 2 layers of the following ingredients into each parfait glass, each layer to go in this order: 2 Tbsp pumpkin mixture, 1 Tbsp whipped topping, 1 layer berries. Garnish the top of the last layer with cinnamon. Chill for 1 hour. Serve

Winter

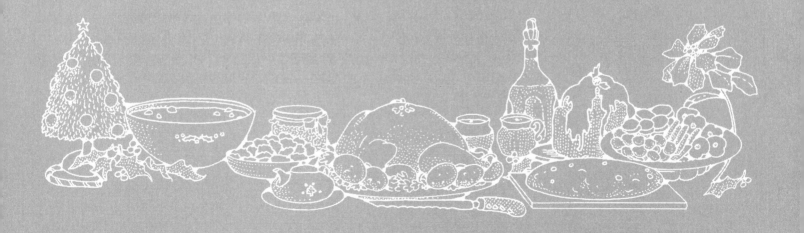

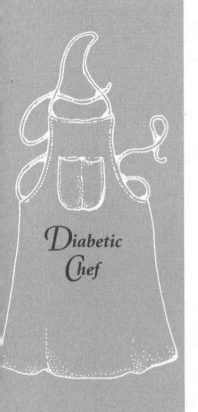

Diabetic Chef

When I think about winter, I am put in mind of heavy sweaters and a warm fire in the hearth. Of holiday shopping and children on vacation. Of the stillness in the air as the snow dances through the sky and blankets the land. Winter is a truly wonderful season.

With winter comes some of our favorite holidays. It is a season for families and friends to gather, to celebrate the blessings we all share. It is also a time to ring in the new year, to reflect on the year past, and to make some resolutions for the future. But no matter what happens, it almost always takes place around the dinner table, where we all gather to celebrate and feast. Food not only nourishes our bodies, it also brings us together and nurtures our souls.

Winter is sometimes a difficult time for finding fresh ingredients. With the miracle of modern shipping, however, many ingredients are available at your local grocery store all year long. It is not unheard of to see asparagus in December, or juicy red tomatoes in March.

I find this time of year best suited to comfort foods. From soups like *Cream of Potato* and *Split Pea*, to casserole dishes like *Chicken Pot Pie* and *Lamb Stew*. These foods are filling and help keep you warm on those cold, snowy nights. They are also easy to prepare, so enjoy!

*B*reakfast Hash Browns

Ingredients

- 1 lb Idaho potatoes, peeled and grated
- 1/2 cup red bell pepper, diced
- 1/2 cup onion, thinly sliced
- 1/2 tsp salt
- 1/4 tsp black pepper
  Nonstick cooking spray

4 Servings

Serving Size: about 2 hash browns

Calories	90
Calories from Fat	2
Total Fat	>1 g
Saturated Fat	0 g
Cholesterol	0 mg
Sodium	1168 mg
Carbohydrate	21 g
Dietary Fiber	2 g
Sugars	3 g
Protein	2 g

Exchanges
1 Starch
1/2 Vegetable

Preparation

1. Combine the potatoes, red bell pepper, onion, salt, and black pepper. Mix well. Spray a pan with nonstick cooking spray and heat over medium heat. Scoop 1/4 cup of the potato mixture into the pan and cook for about 10 minutes, or until the bottom is golden brown. Flip the hash brown and cook the remaining side for 8–10 minutes, or until it is also golden brown. Repeat until all the hash browns are used.

Oatmeal with Cranberry and Brown Sugar

Ingredients

1 1/2 cups oatmeal
   3 cups fat-free (skim) milk
   1 cup dried cranberries
   1 tsp brown sugar
     Pinch cinnamon

4 Servings
Serving Size: about 2/3 cup

Calories	160
Calories from Fat	15
Total Fat	2 g
Saturated Fat	>1 g
Cholesterol	0 mg
Sodium	2 mg
Carbohydrate	31 g
Dietary Fiber	4 g
Sugars	13 g
Protein	4 g

Exchanges
1 Starch
1 Fruit

Preparation

1. Follow the directions for cooking oatmeal on the box, but use the fat-free milk instead of water. When the oatmeal has finished cooking, add the dried cranberries and brown sugar and mix well. Garnish the tops with cinnamon.

Poached Egg with Spicy Red Pepper Puree

Ingredients

4   red bell peppers, diced
1/2 cup white wine
1/3 cup shallots, diced
       Dash hot pepper sauce
1   quart water
2   tsp white vinegar
4   large eggs

4 Servings
Serving Size: 1 egg,
       1/3 cup sauce

Calories	146
Calories from Fat	47
Total Fat	5 g
Saturated Fat	2 g
Cholesterol	213 mg
Sodium	70 mg
Carbohydrate	13 g
Dietary Fiber	2 g
Sugars	5 g
Protein	8 g

Exchanges
1 Lean Meat
2 Vegetable
1 Fat

Preparation

1. Place the red bell peppers, white wine, and shallots in a pan over low heat and cover. Cook for about 25–30 minutes, or until the peppers are very tender. Place the mixture in a food processor and puree until it is smooth. Season it with a dash hot pepper sauce and set it aside.
2. Place the water and vinegar in a shallow pan and bring the liquid to a boil. Reduce the heat to a simmer. Crack one egg into a cup or mug, then pour the egg very gently into the water. Cook the egg for 3–5 minutes. Remove the egg from the water and serve immediately with the red pepper puree overtop. Repeat the process with the remaining eggs.

*P*ecan-Crusted Pork Chops

Ingredients

2 cups pecans, crushed
1 tsp black pepper
4 boneless pork chops, fat
   trimmed
2 large eggs, beaten
   Nonstick cooking spray

4 Servings
Serving Size: 1 pork chop

Calories	616
Calories from Fat	398
Total Fat	44 g
Saturated Fat	6 g
Cholesterol	233 mg
Sodium	102 mg
Carbohydrate	11 g
Dietary Fiber	5 g
Sugars	3 g
Protein	36 g

Exchanges
3 1/2 Very Lean Meat
1 Lean Meat
7 Fat

Preparation

1. Preheat the oven to 350°F. Combine the pecans and black pepper in a small bowl. Dip the pork chops in the egg, then dredge the pork chops through the pecan mixture until they are well coated. Spray a baking sheet with nonstick cooking spray and place the pork chops on it. Bake for 23–35 minutes, or until the pork chops are well done.

*P*ork Tenderloin Wellington

Ingredients

Nonstick cooking
spray
1 lb pork tenderloin,
clean of sinew
1 tsp salt
1 tsp black pepper
1 Tbsp olive oil
1 lb assorted mush-
rooms (white,
Shiitake, Portabello,
oyster, etc.), sliced
1 cup dry sherry
1/4 tsp black pepper
1 sheet puff pastry

6 Servings
Serving Size: 9 oz

Calories	374
Calories from Fat	120
Total Fat	13 g
Saturated Fat	4 g
Cholesterol	134 mg
Sodium	505 mg
Carbohydrate	7 g
Dietary Fiber	1 g
Sugars	2 g
Protein	50 g

Exchanges
7 Very Lean Meat
1 Vegetable
2 Fat

Preparation

1. Preheat the oven to 350°F. Spray a pan with cooking spray and heat over medium heat. Season the tenderloin with the salt and black pepper, then place it into the pan. Brown all sides of the tenderloin, then remove it to a roasting rack. Cook in the oven for about 15–20 minutes, or until the tenderloin reaches an internal temperature of 155°F. Remove from oven and allow to cool 30–45 minutes.

2. Heat the olive oil in a pan over medium heat. Add the mushrooms and cook, stirring frequently, for about 5–6 minutes, or until the mushrooms are tender. Add the dry sherry and scrape the bottom of the pan with the flat end of a spatula. Add the black pepper. Bring the liquid to a simmer and allow it to reduce until the pan is almost dry, about 5–8 minutes. Remove from the heat and allow to cool.

3. Roll the puff pastry sheet out on a counter. Spoon 1 cup of the mushroom mixture onto the bottom third of the pastry. Place the tenderloin on top of the mushroom mixture. Roll the pastry dough with the tenderloin inside and be certain to close the seams at either end of the tenderloin. Make slits about 1 inch apart across the top of the puff pastry. Place into a 350 degree oven and cook until the puff pastry is golden brown, about 45–50 minutes. Let the tenderloin rest for 5–10 minutes before serving.

Chicken Kiev

Ingredients

- 4   boneless, skinless chicken breasts
- 1   tsp salt
- 1/2 tsp white pepper
- 2   Tbsp Herb Butter (see p. 158)
- 1/2 cup all-purpose flour
- 1   large egg, beaten
- 1/2 cup dry bread crumbs
      Nonstick cooking spray

4 Servings
Serving Size:
   1 chicken breast

Calories	**433**
Calories from Fat	117
Total Fat	13 g
Saturated Fat	7 g
Cholesterol	188 mg
Sodium	780 mg
Carbohydrate	13 g
Dietary Fiber	1 g
Sugars	1 g
Protein	31 g

Exchanges
1 Starch
3 1/2 Very Lean Meat
3 Fat

Preparation

1. Preheat the oven to 375°F. Using a mallet or meat tenderizer, pound the chicken breasts until they are very thin. Season the chicken breasts with salt and white pepper. Place 1/2 Tbsp of Herb Butter in the center of each chicken breast, roll the chicken breasts up, and secure the chicken breasts with toothpicks. Make sure there are no openings through which the butter can leak out.
2. Coat the chicken breasts with flour, dip them in the egg, then dredge them through the bread crumbs until each piece is well covered. Spray a pan with nonstick cooking spray and heat over medium heat. Add the rolled breasts and brown on all sides.
3. Bake the browned chicken breasts in the oven for about 15 minutes (internal temperature of 160°F). Serve immediately.

Chicken Pot Pie

Ingredients

Nonstick cooking spray
3/4 cup onion, diced
1/2 cup carrot, diced
1/2 cup celery, diced
2 cups Chicken Stock (see p. 155)
4 boneless, skinless chicken breasts, medium diced
1 1/2 cups potatoes, peeled and diced
1 Tbsp fresh rosemary, finely chopped
1 Tbsp fresh thyme, finely chopped
4 Tbsp cornstarch
6 Tbsp water
Basic Pie Pastry (see p. 151), or use store-bought dough

8 Servings
Serving Size: about 1 cup

Calories	281
Calories from Fat	79
Total Fat	9 g
Saturated Fat	1 g
Cholesterol	37 mg
Sodium	96 mg
Carbohydrate	33 g
Dietary Fiber	2 g
Sugars	6 g
Protein	17 g

Exchanges
2 Starch
2 Lean Meat
1 Vegetable
1 1/2 Fat

Preparation

1. Preheat the oven to 400°F. Spray a large pot with nonstick cooking spray and heat over medium heat. Add the onions, carrots, and celery and cook about 5–6 minutes, or until the vegetables are almost tender. Add the chicken stock and bring the liquid to a simmer. Add the chicken and potatoes and return the liquid to a simmer. Cook for 25 minutes. Add the rosemary and thyme.

2. In a separate bowl, mix the cornstarch and water until it forms a smooth paste. Stir the cornstarch mixture into the pot. Return the liquid to a simmer for 5 minutes. Place the mixture in a 8 × 8-inch casserole dish, cover with the pastry dough, and bake for 30 minutes, or until the crust is golden brown.

Curry Chicken

Ingredients

1 whole chicken, cut into
  8 pieces
1 tsp salt
1 tsp black pepper
2 Tbsp curry powder
1 Tbsp olive oil
1 medium onion, diced
1 medium carrot, diced
1 cup white wine
2 cups Chicken Stock (see
  p. 155)

4 Servings
Serving Size: 2 pieces
  of chicken

Calories	282
Calories from Fat	194
Total Fat	22 g
Saturated Fat	2 g
Cholesterol	15 mg
Sodium	611 mg
Carbohydrate	7 g
Dietary Fiber	2 g
Sugars	2 g
Protein	2 g

Exchanges
3 1/2 Lean Meat
1 Vegetable
3 1/2 Fat

Preparation

1. Wash the cut chicken pieces and pat dry with a paper towel. Combine the salt, black pepper, and curry powder and rub into the chicken pieces. Cover the chicken and allow it to refrigerate overnight.
2. Preheat the oven to 375°F. Heat the olive oil in a pan over medium-high heat. Add the chicken and cook, turning frequently, until the chicken is seared on all sides. Place the chicken on a baking sheet and bake for 20 minutes.
3. Using the same pan used for the chicken, lower the heat to medium and add the onion and carrot. Cook for 5–6 minutes, or until the vegetables are tender. Add the white wine, bring the liquid to a simmer, and allow it to reduce until the pan is almost dry. Add the chicken stock and return the liquid to a simmer. Add the chicken pieces to the pan and cook for 5 minutes. The curry from the chicken will thicken the sauce. Serve immediately.

Poached Cornish Game Hen with Baby Vegetables and Orzo Pasta

Ingredients

2 Cornish game hens
1 tsp salt
2 tsp black pepper
1 Tbsp olive oil
1 Tbsp fresh rosemary, chopped
1 Tbsp fresh chives, chopped
1 Tbsp fresh thyme, chopped
1 Tbsp fresh oregano, chopped
2 cups pearl onions
2 cups baby carrots
2 cups white wine
1 quart Chicken Stock (see p. 155)
2 cups zucchini, sliced and quartered
1 cup frozen peas
2 quarts water
1 cup orzo pasta

4 Servings

Serving Size: 1/2 hen, 1 cup pasta, 2/3 cup vegetables and stock

Calories	368
Calories from Fat	115
Total Fat	13 g
Saturated Fat	3 g
Cholesterol	67 mg
Sodium	550 mg
Carbohydrate	29 g
Dietary Fiber	2 g
Sugars	4 g
Protein	26 g

Exchanges

1 1/2 Starch
3 Lean Meat
1 1/2 Vegetable
1 1/2 Fat

Preparation

1. Truss each Cornish game hen by tying the legs together with butcher's twine. Rub the salt, black pepper, and olive oil into the skin of each hen. Combine the rosemary, chives, thyme, and oregano in a bowl and set aside.
2. Heat a large pot over medium-high heat and place the Cornish game hens inside. Brown all sides of the game hens. Add the pearl onions and baby carrots and cook for 2–3 minutes. Add the white wine and scrape the bottom of the pot with the flat end of a spatula. Allow the liquid to reduce until the pot is almost dry. Add the chicken stock and bring the liquid to a simmer. Cook the game hens in the liquid for 1 hour.
3. Add the zucchini to the pot and cook for another 10 minutes. Add the peas and cook for 5 minutes. Remove the pot from the heat.
4. Remove hen from pot. Using a sharp knife, carefully slice from the breast bone lengthwise down the breast, keeping the knife next to the bone. With the tip of the knife, follow through around the underside of the hen. Now, still using the tip of the knife, cut the breast away from the rest of the hen. Finally, cut the leg and thigh piece away.
5. While the hens are being poached, bring the 2 quarts of water to a boil in a separate pot. Add the orzo pasta and cook for 10–12 minutes, or until the pasta is done.
6. Serve the Cornish game hens in a bowl with 1 cup of the pasta, 1 Tbsp of the fresh herbs, and 2/3 cup of the chicken stock with the baby vegetables.

*S*autéed Duck Breast with Raspberry Glaze

Ingredients

- 4 duck breasts, skin on
- 1/2 tsp salt
- 1 tsp black pepper
- 1 Tbsp olive oil
- 1/2 pint fresh raspberries, pureed and strained of seeds
- 1/2 lemon, juiced

4 Servings
Serving Size: 1 duck breast

Calories	304
Calories from Fat	151
Total Fat	17 g
Saturated Fat	4 g
Cholesterol	163 mg
Sodium	392 mg
Carbohydrate	8 g
Dietary Fiber	4 g
Sugars	3 g
Protein	30 g

Exchanges
4 Lean Meat
1/2 Fruit
1 Fat

Preparation

1. Preheat the oven to 375°F. Season the duck breasts with the salt and pepper. Heat the olive oil in a pan over medium-high heat. Add the duck breasts, skin down, to the pan and allow the skin to sear to a golden brown, about 6–8 minutes. Turn the duck breasts over and sear remaining side to golden brown, about 2–4 minutes.
2. Brush each duck breast with the raspberry puree. Bake the duck breasts in the oven for about 10–15 minutes, or until they reach an internal temperature of 165°F. Be sure to brush the breasts with the raspberry puree every 5 minutes.
3. Serve each duck breast brushed with the raspberry puree and sprinkled with lemon juice.

*V*eal Osso Buco

Ingredients

 2 veal shanks, cut in half
    lengthwise
 1 tsp salt
 2 tsp black pepper
1/2 cup all-purpose flour
 2 Tbsp olive oil
 2 cups onion, chopped
 1 cup carrots, chopped
 1 cup celery, chopped
 2 cups white wine
 1 16-oz can crushed
    tomatoes
 2 Tbsp garlic, crushed
 4 cups low-sodium beef
    broth
 1 sprig fresh rosemary
 2 sprigs fresh thyme
 4 bay leaves

8 Servings
Serving Size: 1/4 veal
    shank, 1 cup sauce

Calories	262
Calories from Fat	64
Total Fat	7 g
Saturated Fat	2 g
Cholesterol	94 mg
Sodium	467 mg
Carbohydrate	14 g
Dietary Fiber	3 g
Sugars	4 g
Protein	29 g

Exchanges
4 Very Lean Meat
2 Vegetable
1 1/2 Fat

Preparation

1. Preheat the oven to 400°F. Place a roasting pan in the oven to heat it. Season the veal with salt and pepper, then dredge the veal through the flour until it is well coated. Add olive oil to the heated roasting pan, then add the veal shanks, onion, carrot, and celery. Bake for 15 minutes, then turn the shanks over and bake for another 15 minutes. This will allow the shanks to brown on all sides.
2. Remove the roasting pan from the oven and add the white wine to it. Lower the oven temperature to 325°F and add the rest of the ingredients to the roasting pan (keep the rosemary, thyme, and bay leaves in a cheesecloth). Bake for 2 hours, tightly covered.
3. Discard the herbs, remove the veal shanks from the roasting pan, and puree the rest of the pan's contents in a food processor. Cut the veal shanks in two and serve each portion with 1/2 cup of the puree as a sauce.

*L*amb Stew

Ingredients

1/2 lb lean-cut lamb, cut into 3/4-inch cubes
1/2 tsp salt
1/4 tsp pepper
3 Tbsp all-purpose flour
1 Tbsp olive oil
3/4 cup onion, diced
1/2 cup carrots, diced
1/2 cup celery, diced
1/2 cup dry red wine (such as Merlot)
1/2 cup turnips, peeled and diced
1 cups potatoes, peeled and diced
1 Tbsp garlic, minced
2 cups low-sodium beef broth
1 Tbsp ground cumin
1 Tbsp cornstarch
1/4 cup water
2 Tbsp parsley leaves, finely chopped

5 Servings
Serving Size: about 1 cup

Calories	186
Calories from Fat	55
Total Fat	6 g
Saturated Fat	2 g
Cholesterol	31 mg
Sodium	310 mg
Carbohydrate	16 g
Dietary Fiber	2 g
Sugars	3 g
Protein	13 g

Exchanges
1 Starch
2 Very Lean Meat
1 Fat

Preparation

1. Season the lamb with the salt and pepper, then dredge through the flour until the lamb pieces are well coated. Heat half the olive oil in a large pot over medium heat. Add the lamb and brown the pieces on all sides. Do not fully cook. Remove the lamb from the pot and set aside.

2. Add the rest of the olive oil, the onion, the carrots, and the celery to the pot. Cook about 5 minutes, or until the vegetables are tender. Remove the vegetables and set aside.

3. Add the red wine and scrape the bottom of the pot with the flat edge of a spatula. Bring the wine to a simmer and allow it to reduce by half. Add the turnips, potatoes, garlic, beef broth, cumin, and lamb pieces. Bring the liquid to a simmer for 30 minutes. Add the cooked vegetables and continue to simmer for 30 minutes more.

4. In a separate bowl, mix the cornstarch with the water until it forms a smooth paste. Slowly stir the cornstarch into the pot until the stew begins to thicken. Simmer for 5 minutes, then serve with a garnish of chopped parsley.

Rosemary Pork Roast

Ingredients

- 1 4-lb boneless pork shoulder blade roast
- 2 sprigs fresh rosemary
- 1 Tbsp olive oil
- 1 tsp salt
- 1 tsp black pepper
- 1 cup Chicken Stock (see p. 155)
- 3 Tbsp cornstarch
- 1/4 cup water

12 Servings
Serving Size: 1 slice pork, 2 Tbsp gravy

Calories	384
Calories from Fat	261
Total Fat	29 g
Saturated Fat	11 g
Cholesterol	106 mg
Sodium	228 mg
Carbohydrate	2 g
Dietary Fiber	0 g
Sugars	0 g
Protein	27 g

Exchanges
4 Lean Meat
3 1/2 Fat

Preparation

1. Preheat the oven to 325°F. Have your butcher or grocery store tie the roast so that it will not come undone in the oven. With a sharp knife, slice a narrow slit between the layer of fat and the meat on both sides. Place a sprig of rosemary in each slit. Rub the olive oil, salt, and black pepper into the meat.
2. Place the roast in the oven for 1 1/2–2 hours, or until the roast reaches an internal temperature of 170°F. Remove the roast from the pan and allow it to cool.
3. Scrape drippings from the roasting pan into a separate bowl. Add the chicken stock and mix. Spoon out any of the fat. Bring the remaining liquid to a simmer on the stove.
4. In a separate bowl, mix the cornstarch and water until it forms a smooth paste. Slowly stir the cornstarch mixture into the liquid until it thickens. Strain the liquid and serve it as a gravy for the pork.

Black Bean and Orzo Pasta

Ingredients

- 4 oz black beans, dried
- 1/2 Tbsp olive oil
- 1/2 cup onion, diced
- 1/2 red bell pepper, diced
- 1/2 Tbsp garlic, minced
- 1/2 cup cooking sherry
- 2 cups Chicken Stock (see p. 155)
- 1 1/2 quarts water
- 1/2 tsp salt
- 4 oz orzo pasta
- 1/2 Tbsp fresh oregano, chopped
- 1/2 Tbsp fresh thyme, chopped
- 1/2 tsp fresh rosemary, chopped
- 1/2 tsp salt
- 1/2 tsp black pepper
- 2 green onions, chopped

5 Servings
Serving Size: 1/2 cup

Calories	201
Calories from Fat	19
Total Fat	2 g
Saturated Fat	0 g
Cholesterol	0 mg
Sodium	380 mg
Carbohydrate	33 g
Dietary Fiber	6 g
Sugars	3 g
Protein	8 g

Exchanges
2 Starch
1/2 Vegetable
1/2 Fat

Preparation

1. Place the black beans in water, cover, and soak overnight.
2. Heat the olive oil in a pot over medium heat. Add the onions, red bell pepper, and garlic. Cook until the onion is translucent, about 5 minutes. Add the cooking sherry and allow it reduce until the pan is almost dry.
3. Add the chicken stock and the drained black beans. Bring the liquid to a boil, lower the heat to a simmer, and cook for 1 1/2 hours, or until the beans are tender. Add more chicken stock if needed.
4. Bring the 3 quarts of water to a boil. Add the salt and pasta and stir to prevent the pasta from sticking. Cook for 10–12 minutes, or until the pasta is done.
5. And the pasta to the pot of black beans. Add the oregano, thyme, and rosemary. Return to a simmer. Season with salt and pepper and serve with chopped green onions on the top.

Chef's Hints: When storing dried beans, always keep them in a cool, dry place. Beans will last for up to a year if stored in their unopened bag or in a sealed container. Never mix old and new beans together because the cooking times might vary.

*L*inguine with Roasted Red Pepper Sauce

Ingredients

2 medium red bell peppers
1/4 cup white wine
1/4 cup shallots, chopped
Dash hot pepper sauce
1 lb linguine pasta, cooked

4 Servings
Serving Size: 1 cup pasta, 1/2 cup sauce

Calories	187
Calories from Fat	12
Total Fat	1 g
Saturated Fat	0 g
Cholesterol	0 mg
Sodium	104 mg
Carbohydrate	37 g
Dietary Fiber	2 g
Sugars	3 g
Protein	7 g

Exchanges
2 Starch
1 Vegetable

Preparation

1. Place the red bell peppers directly on the burners of a gas stove and turn the heat on high. Allow the skin to turn completely black, turning the pepper occasionally. When all the peppers are blackened, put them in a large bowl and cover with plastic wrap to steam the skins away. After 10 minutes, run the peppers under cold water and peel away the skins. Remove the tops and seeds of the peppers and roughly chop.
2. Place the red peppers, white wine, and shallots in a pan over high heat. Bring the mixture to a boil, then reduce the heat to a simmer for 20 minutes.
3. Place the red pepper mixture into a food processor and puree. If the sauce is too thick, add some hot chicken stock (see p. 155). Add a dash hot pepper sauce, mix well, and serve over cooked pasta.

*L*inguine with Roasted Yellow Pepper Sauce

Ingredients

- 2 medium yellow bell peppers
- 1/4 cup white wine
- 1/4 cup shallots, chopped
- 1/4 tsp white pepper
- 1 lb linguine pasta, cooked

4 Servings

Serving Size: 1 cup pasta, 1/2 cup sauce

Calories	196
Calories from Fat	13
Total Fat	1 g
Saturated Fat	0 g
Cholesterol	0 mg
Sodium	105 mg
Carbohydrate	39 g
Dietary Fiber	3 g
Sugars	4 g
Protein	7 g

Exchanges

2 Starch
1 Vegetable

Preparation

1. Place the yellow bell peppers directly on the burners of a gas stove and turn the heat on high. Allow the skin to turn completely black, turning the pepper occasionally. When all the peppers are blackened, put them in a large bowl and cover with plastic wrap to steam the skins away. After 10 minutes, run the peppers under cold water and peel away the skins. Remove the tops and seeds of the peppers and roughly chop.
2. Place the yellow peppers, white wine, and shallots in a pan over high heat. Bring the mixture to a boil, then reduce the heat to a simmer for 20 minutes.
3. Place the yellow pepper mixture into a food processor and puree. If the sauce is too thick, add some hot chicken stock (see p. 155). Add the white pepper, mix well, and serve over cooked pasta.

*L*inguine with Pesto Sauce

Ingredients

- 1   cup fresh basil, without stems, chopped
- 1/4 cup toasted pine nuts
- 1   tsp garlic, minced
- 3/4 cup extra virgin olive oil
- 1/4 tsp pepper
- 1   lb linguine pasta, cooked

4 Servings

Serving Size: 1 cup pasta, 1/2 cup pesto

Calories	487
Calories from Fat	313
Total Fat	35 g
Saturated Fat	6 g
Cholesterol	4 mg
Sodium	220 mg
Carbohydrate	36 g
Dietary Fiber	4 g
Sugars	1 g
Protein	12 g

Exchanges

2 Starch
1 Lean Meat
1/2 Vegetable
6 Fat

Preparation

1. Put the basil, pine nuts, and garlic into a food processor on medium speed. Slowly drizzle the olive oil into the food processor while it is running. Turn the food processor off, add the black pepper, and mix well. Serve over cooked linguine.

Linguine with Trio of Sauces

Ingredients

- 2 cups Roasted Red Pepper Sauce (from p. 125)
- 2 cups Roasted Yellow Pepper Sauce (from p. 126)
- 2 cups Pesto Sauce (from p. 127)
- 1 lb linguine pasta, cooked
- 1/4 cup Parmesan cheese, grated

4 Servings
Serving Size: 1/3 cup of pasta from each sauce

Calories	488
Calories from Fat	250
Total Fat	28 g
Saturated Fat	5 g
Cholesterol	4 mg
Sodium	101 mg
Carbohydrate	46 g
Dietary Fiber	5 g
Sugars	4 g
Protein	12 g

Exchanges
2 Starch
1/2 Lean Meat
2 Vegetables
5 Fat

Preparation

1. Divide the pasta into thirds. Dip each third of pasta into separate bowls of the Roasted Red Pepper, Roasted Yellow Pepper, and Pesto sauces. Twirl the pasta well in each sauce. Arrange a sampling of pasta that has been dipped in each sauce on every plate so that the pastas appear to be three different nests. Garnish with Parmesan cheese and serve.

Baked Halibut with Lemon Dill Sauce

Ingredients

- 4   halibut steaks, 1-inch thick
- 2   Tbsp water
- 1   Tbsp lemon rind, grated
- 1   Tbsp fresh dill, chopped
- 1   Tbsp balsamic vinegar
- 1   Tbsp onion, diced
- 1/2   tsp garlic, minced
- 2 1/2   Tbsp olive oil
- 1/8   tsp salt
- 1/8   tsp pepper

4 Servings

Serving Size: 1 halibut steak, 2 Tbsp sauce

Calories	367
Calories from Fat	267
Total Fat	30 g
Saturated Fat	5 g
Cholesterol	71 mg
Sodium	125 mg
Carbohydrate	1 g
Dietary Fiber	0 g
Sugars	1 g
Protein	22 g

Exchanges

3 1/2 Very Lean Meat
5 1/2 Fat

Preparation

1. Preheat the oven to 350°F. Bake the halibut steaks for 15–20 minutes, or until the fish is fully cooked and flaky.
2. In a separate bowl, mix together the remaining ingredients. Serve over finished halibut steaks.

Baked Spanish Mackerel with Tomato Caper Sauce

Ingredients

1 lemon
4 Spanish mackerel filets, cleaned and bones removed
1 tsp black pepper
4 tsp Herb Butter (see p. 158)
1 Tbsp olive oil
1 Tbsp garlic, minced
2 Tbsp onion, diced
1 cup white wine
4 medium tomatoes, skinned, seeded, and diced
1 Tbsp capers
   Pinch black pepper
2 Tbsp fresh basil, chopped

4 Servings
Serving Size: 1 filet,
   1 cup sauce

Calories	370
Calories from Fat	152
Total Fat	17 g
Saturated Fat	6 g
Cholesterol	117 mg
Sodium	191 mg
Carbohydrate	10 g
Dietary Fiber	2 g
Sugars	4 g
Protein	36 g

Exchanges
4 Very Lean Meat
1 Vegetable
3 1/2 Fat

Preparation

1. Preheat the oven to 350°F. Grate the lemon rind. Season the filets with the black pepper and the lemon rind. Roll the filets from the end and secure with a toothpick so that the filet will not unroll in the oven. Place 1 tsp of Herb Butter on top of each filet. Squeeze lemon juice over the filets. Bake for 20–25 minutes, or until the fish is fully cooked.

2. Heat the olive oil in a pan over medium heat. Add the garlic and onion and cook for 5 minutes, or until the onion is translucent. Add the white wine and allow the liquid to reduce by half.

3. Add the tomatoes and cook 10 minutes, or until the tomatoes are very tender. Add the capers and cook 5 more minutes. Remove from the heat. Add the black pepper and basil and serve overtop the filets.

Sautéed Calamari with Roasted Fennel Cream Sauce and Angel Hair Pasta

Ingredients

- 1 fennel bulb
- 1/2 Tbsp olive oil
- 1/4 tsp black pepper
- 1/2 Tbsp sugar
- 1 cup evaporated skim milk
- 1/2 lb calamari, sliced into strips or rings
- 1/2 tsp salt
- 1/4 tsp black pepper
- 1/2 tsp garlic powder
- 1/4 tsp red pepper flakes
- 1/4 cup all-purpose flour
- 1/2 Tbsp olive oil
- 3/4 lb angel hair pasta
- 2 quarts boiling water

4 Servings

Serving Size: 2/3 cup pasta, 1/4 sauce

Calories	474
Calories from Fat	73
Total Fat	8 g
Saturated Fat	2 g
Cholesterol	12 mg
Sodium	544 mg
Carbohydrate	79 g
Dietary Fiber	3 g
Sugars	52 g
Protein	23 g

Exchanges

5 Starch
1 Lean Meat
1/2 Vegetable
1 Fat

Preparation

1. Cut the top stems from the fennel, then slice the fennel in half lengthwise to expose the core. Remove the core and discard, then cut the fennel into very thin strips.
2. Heat the olive oil in a pan over medium heat. Add the fennel to the pan and do not stir. Once the fennel turns brown on one side, turn it over and allow it to brown on the other side. Add the black pepper and sugar and toss to coat. Add the evaporated skim milk and bring the liquid to a simmer. Remove from the heat and set aside.
3. Mix the calamari with the salt, black pepper, garlic powder, red pepper flakes, and flour until well coated. Heat the olive oil in a pan over medium-high heat. Add the calamari and cook 2–3 minutes, or until done. Add the calamari to the fennel sauce.
4. In a large pot, bring the water to a boil. Add the angel hair pasta and stir frequently to prevent the pasta from sticking. Cook for 8–10 minutes, or until the pasta is done. Serve the pasta topped with the calamari and fennel sauce.

*S*picy Shrimp with Dijon Sauce and Linguine

Ingredients

1/2 lb shrimp, deveined
    and without shells
1 Tbsp paprika
1 tsp garlic powder
1/2 tsp cayenne pepper
1 tsp onion powder
1 tsp thyme
1/2 tsp black pepper
1 tsp olive oil
1/4 cup onion, diced
1/2 Tbsp garlic, minced
1/4 cup tomatoes, diced
1/8 cup white wine
1/4 cup Dijon mustard
1/2 cup Chicken Stock
    (see p. 155)
1 lb linguine pasta,
    cooked

4 Servings

Serving Size: 1/2 cup pasta,
    1/4 sauce with shrimp

Calories	271
Calories from Fat	17
Total Fat	2 g
Saturated Fat	0 g
Cholesterol	81 mg
Sodium	166 mg
Carbohydrate	45 g
Dietary Fiber	3 g
Sugars	2 g
Protein	16 g

Exchanges

3 Starch
1 Very Lean Meat

Preparation

1. Combine the shrimp with the paprika, garlic powder, cayenne pepper, onion powder, thyme, and black pepper. Toss until well coated. Cover and refrigerate for 1 hour.
2. Heat half the olive oil in a pan over medium-high heat. Add the shrimp and cook, stirring constantly, for 3–5 minutes, or until the shrimp turn pink and are firm to the touch. Remove from pan and set aside.
3. Add the rest of the olive oil, the onion, and the garlic. Cook for about 3 minutes, or until the onion is translucent. Add the tomatoes and white wine. Let the liquid reduce until the pan is almost dry. Add the Dijon mustard and chicken stock. Bring the liquid to a simmer and allow it to reduce by one-half.
4. Serve the sauce with the shrimp overtop the pasta.

Tinfoil-Wrapped Swordfish Steak

Ingredients

4 swordfish steaks, about
    6 oz each
4 oz Herb Butter
    (see p. 158)
1 lemon, thinly sliced
4 sprigs fresh dill
1 Tbsp fresh rosemary,
    chopped
1 tsp black pepper

4 Servings
Serving Size:
    1 swordfish steak

Calories	347
Calories from Fat	250
Total Fat	28 g
Saturated Fat	16 g
Cholesterol	107 mg
Sodium	108 mg
Carbohydrate	1 g
Dietary Fiber	0 g
Sugars	0 g
Protein	23 g

Exchanges
3 1/2 Very Lean Meat
5 Fat

Preparation

1. Preheat the oven to 350°F. Lay each swordfish steak on a piece of aluminum foil. Place 1 oz of Herb Butter on each swordfish steak. Lay 2 slices of lemon and 1 sprig of dill on top. Season each steak with the rosemary and black pepper. Bring the two ends of the foil together and fold into a tight seam. Roll this seam three times, then fold in the loose ends.
2. Bake in the oven for 25–30 minutes, or until the fish is fully cooked and firm to the touch. Serve immediately.

Chef's Hint: To keep food from over-browning, wrap the food in aluminum foil with the shiny side out.

Cream of Potato Soup

Ingredients

1/2 Tbsp olive oil
1/2 medium onion, diced
1 stalk celery, diced
1 quart Chicken Stock (see p. 155)
1 lb potatoes, peeled and quartered
1/2 tsp marjoram
1/2 tsp thyme
1 cup low-fat (1%) milk
1/2 tsp salt
1/4 tsp white pepper
4 Tbsp fresh parsley, minced

6 Servings
Serving Size: about 1 cup

Calories	121
Calories from Fat	27
Total Fat	3 g
Saturated Fat	1 g
Cholesterol	6 mg
Sodium	296 mg
Carbohydrate	19 g
Dietary Fiber	2 g
Sugars	4 g
Protein	5 g

Exchanges
1 Starch
1/2 Fat

Preparation

1. Heat the olive oil in a large pot over medium heat. Add the onion and celery and cook about 5 minutes, or until the vegetables are tender. Add the chicken stock, potatoes, marjoram, and thyme. Bring to a simmer and cover to cook for 25–30 minutes, or until the potatoes are tender.
2. Place the mixture in a food processor and blend until smooth. Whisk in the milk until the mixture is thin enough. Add the salt and pepper and mix well. Serve with 1 Tbsp of parsley overtop of each bowl.

Split Pea Soup

Ingredients

1/2 slice bacon, diced
1/2 medium onion, diced
1/4 medium carrot, diced
1/4 stalk celery, diced
 1 tsp garlic, minced
1/4 tsp thyme
1/3 tsp marjoram
1/4 lb split peas, dried
 3 cups Chicken Stock
    (see p. 155)
1/4 tsp salt
1/8 tsp white pepper

4 Servings
Serving Size: about 1 cup

Calories	131
Calories from Fat	28
Total Fat	3 g
Saturated Fat	1 g
Cholesterol	5 mg
Sodium	254 mg
Carbohydrate	18 g
Dietary Fiber	6 g
Sugars	4 g
Protein	9 g

Exchanges
1 Starch
1/2 Lean Meat
1/2 Fat

Preparation

1. Heat a medium pot over medium heat. Add the bacon, cook, and render the fat. Add the onion, carrot, celery, and garlic and cook for 5 minutes, or until the vegetables are tender. Add the thyme, marjoram, split peas, and chicken stock. Bring to a simmer and cover for 1 1/2–2 hours, stirring occasionally to prevent burning on the bottom of the pot.
2. Pour the mixture into a food processor and blend until smooth. Add the salt and white pepper and mix well.

Watercress and Endive Salad with Apple Cider Vinaigrette

Ingredients

1 1/4 cups pine nuts
5 Tbsp cider vinegar
8 Tbsp olive oil
1/4 Granny Smith apple, cored and diced
1/2 shallot, minced
Pinch black pepper
2 endives, cored and leaves separated
12 oz watercress
2 Tbsp fresh chives, chopped

4 Servings
Serving Size: 1/4 recipe

Calories	274
Calories from Fat	211
Total Fat	23 g
Saturated Fat	4 g
Cholesterol	0 mg
Sodium	59 mg
Carbohydrate	9 g
Dietary Fiber	5 g
Sugars	2 g
Protein	13 g

Exchanges
1 Very Lean Meat
1/2 Vegetable
4 Fat

Preparation

1. Preheat the oven to 300°F. Place the pine nuts on a baking sheet and bake for 10 minutes, or until they are lightly browned. Remove from the oven and set aside.
2. Place the cider vinegar in a small bowl. Slowly whisk in the olive oil until it is well combined. Stir in the apples, shallots, and black pepper.
3. Place 4 endive leaves on each plate at the 3, 6, 9, and 12 o'clock positions. Place a good handful of endive and watercress in the center of the plate. Drizzle the vinaigrette over the watercress and endive. Garnish with the chives and pine nuts and serve.

Did You Know? Tomatoes, cucumbers, and carrots are the most popular salad items. But that doesn't mean they are the only ingredients. Try this interesting variation.

Roast Beef with Roasted Garlic and Rosemary Gravy

Ingredients

1 3–4 lb boneless beef roast
1 tsp salt
2 tsp black pepper
1 Tbsp olive oil
   Nonstick cooking spray
1 medium onion, diced
1 medium carrot, chopped
1 celery stalk, chopped
1 garlic bulb
1 tsp olive oil
2 cups low-sodium beef broth
1/2 fresh rosemary sprig, minced
2 Tbsp cornstarch
4 Tbsp water

10 Servings
Serving Size: 1 slice with 1/4 cup gravy

Calories	239
Calories from Fat	80
Total Fat	9 g
Saturated Fat	3 g
Cholesterol	94 mg
Sodium	301 mg
Carbohydrate	8 g
Dietary Fiber	2 g
Sugars	0 g
Protein	30 g

Exchanges
3 1/2 Lean Meat
1/2 Fat

Preparation

1. Pre-heat the oven to 325°F. Rub the salt and pepper over the surface of the roast. Pour the olive oil over the meat and rub the olive oil into the surface. Spray a pan with the nonstick cooking spray and place over medium-high heat. Place the beef in the pan and cook until the surface is golden brown, turning the meat as needed until the entire surface is cooked.

2. Place the onions, carrots, and celery at the bottom of a roasting pan. Place the beef on top of the vegetables. Put the entire pan into the oven and cook for 1 hour 45 minutes to 2 hours 15 minutes, or until the meat reaches an internal temperature of 145°F.

3. While the beef is in the oven, prepare your roasted garlic. Slice the top of the garlic bulb so that the garlic pieces are just exposed. Place the bulb on a small baking dish and rub 1 tsp of olive oil over the skin. Put the garlic in the same oven as the beef and bake for 20 minutes, or until the garlic bulb is soft to the touch. Remove the garlic and allow it to cool.

4. Once cool, break open the garlic bulb and squeeze the garlic pulp from the skin. Discard any of the skin or peel. Puree the roasted garlic in a food processor until it is a paste.

5. When the roast is finished, remove the beef from the roasting pan and allow it to cool for 10 minutes. Place the pan with the remaining ingredients over medium heat on the stove top. Add the beef broth and minced rosemary. Stir the pan, making sure to loosen any of the drippings at the bottom. Strain this liquid into a smaller pot and add 1 Tbsp of the roasted garlic puree. Bring the liquid to a simmer.

6. In a separate bowl, mix the cornstarch with the water until it forms a smooth paste. Slowly pour the cornstarch mixture into the simmering liquid, and whisk until the gravy thickens. Slice the beef and serve with gravy on top.

Sun-Dried Tomato and Herb Couscous

Ingredients

- 1 Tbsp olive oil
- 1 cup sun-dried tomatoes, reconstituted in water
- 1/4 red onion, diced
- 2 tsp garlic, chopped
- 2 cups Chicken Stock (see p. 155)
- 4 Tbsp water
- 2 cups couscous
- 1 Tbsp fresh oregano, chopped
- 1 Tbsp fresh basil, chopped
- 1 tsp fresh rosemary, chopped
- 2 tsp fresh thyme, chopped

4 Servings
Serving Size: about 3/4 cup

Calories	403
Calories from Fat	40
Total Fat	4 g
Saturated Fat	1 g
Cholesterol	0 mg
Sodium	296 mg
Carbohydrate	77 g
Dietary Fiber	6 g
Sugars	5 g
Protein	14 g

Exchanges
4 Starch
1 1/2 Vegetable
1 Fat

Preparation

1. Heat the olive oil in a medium pot over medium heat. Add the sun-dried tomatoes, onion, and garlic. Cook until the onions are translucent, about 3–4 minutes. Add the chicken stock and water and bring to a boil. Add the remaining ingredients and stir well.
2. Remove the pot from the heat, cover tightly, and allow it to sit for 10–15 minutes, or until all the water has been absorbed. Fluff with a fork and serve.

Green Beans with Lemon Pepper

Ingredients

1 Tbsp red peppercorns
1 Tbsp green peppercorns
1 tsp black peppercorns
1 tsp white peppercorns
2 lemon rinds, grated
2 quarts water
1 lb fresh green beans
1 tsp salt
1 lemon, cut into 4 wedges

4 Servings
Serving Size: 1/4 recipe

Calories	51
Calories from Fat	7
Total Fat	>1 g
Saturated Fat	0 g
Cholesterol	0 mg
Sodium	586 mg
Carbohydrate	11 g
Dietary Fiber	5 g
Sugars	2 g
Protein	3 g

Exchanges
1 1/2 Vegetable

Preparation

1. Grind the peppercorns in a coffee grinder until they are fine. Add the grated lemon rind and mix well.
2. Bring the water to a boil. Add the green beans and salt. Cook for 5 minutes, or until the beans are tender. Drain and season with 2 Tbsp of the lemon pepper per serving. Serve the green beans with a lemon wedge garnish.

Orange and Honey Glazed Baby Carrots

Ingredients

- 2 tsp butter
- 1 1/2 cup water
- 3/4 lb baby carrots
- 1 cup orange juice
- 1 Tbsp honey
- Pinch white pepper

4 Servings

Serving Size: about 1/2 cup

Calories	93
Calories from Fat	22
Total Fat	3 g
Saturated Fat	1 g
Cholesterol	5 mg
Sodium	31 mg
Carbohydrate	18 g
Dietary Fiber	2 g
Sugars	15 g
Protein	1 g

Exchanges
1/2 Fruit
1 1/2 Vegetable
1/2 Fat

Preparation

1. In a large pan, bring the butter and water to a boil over high heat. Add the carrots and reduce the heat to a simmer. Allow the water to reduce by half, then add the orange juice and honey. Continue to simmer for 10–12 minutes, or until the carrots are tender. Remove the carrots and set aside.
2. Raise the heat and reduce the liquid to about 1/2 cup. The liquid should be thick. Return the carrots to the pan and toss with the liquid. Season with white pepper and serve.

Did You Know? Commercially grown oranges from Florida date back to 1820. Frozen orange juice was not invented until 1940.

$\mathcal{P}$eas and Pearl Onions

Ingredients

- 1 Tbsp olive oil
- 1 8-oz package of frozen pearl onions
- 1 tsp black pepper
- 1/2 cup sherry
- 1 quart water
- 1 8-oz package of frozen peas
- 1 tsp salt

4 Servings
Serving Size: about 2/3 cup

Calories	124
Calories from Fat	33
Total Fat	4 g
Saturated Fat	>1 g
Cholesterol	0 mg
Sodium	210 mg
Carbohydrate	15 g
Dietary Fiber	4 g
Sugars	6 g
Protein	4 g

Exchanges
1/2 Starch
1 Vegetable
1 Fat

Preparation

1. Heat the olive oil in a pan over medium heat. Add the pearl onions and cook until golden brown, about 5–7 minutes. Season with pepper and add the sherry. Reduce the liquid until the pan is almost dry
2. Bring the water to a boil in a separate pot. Add the peas and salt and cook for 3–5 minutes. Drain the peas, add to the pearl onions, and mix well.

Did You Know? Americans have reduced their purchases of fresh vegetables by 12%, increasing the purchases of frozen or canned vegetables by 50%. Canned or frozen vegetables may contain lower healthy enzymes. Fresh is better. Try using fresh peas instead of frozen, if you can.

Buttery String Beans

Ingredients

1/2 lb fresh green beans
  1 quart water
1/2 tsp salt
1/2 Tbsp Herb Butter
    (see p. 158)

4 Servings
Serving Size: 1/4 recipe

Calories	33
Calories from Fat	15
Total Fat	2 g
Saturated Fat	1 g
Cholesterol	4 mg
Sodium	73 mg
Carbohydrate	4 g
Dietary Fiber	2 g
Sugars	1 g
Protein	1 g

Exchanges
1 Vegetable

Preparation

1. Rinse the green beans well in cold water. Remove the tips. Bring the water to a boil. Add the salt and beans, then lower the heat to a light boil. Cook for 3–5 minutes, or until the beans are tender. Drain.
2. Toss the beans with the Herb Butter until the butter has melted. Serve.

*R*oasted Garlic Mashed Potatoes

Ingredients

1   lb potatoes, peeled and quartered
2   quarts water
1/4   cup low-fat (1%) milk
1/2   tsp salt
1/4   tsp white pepper
1 1/2   Tbsp Roasted Garlic Puree (see p. 160)

4 Servings
Serving Size: 5 oz

Calories	104
Calories from Fat	11
Total Fat	1 g
Saturated Fat	1 g
Cholesterol	4 mg
Sodium	422 mg
Carbohydrate	20 g
Dietary Fiber	2 g
Sugars	4 g
Protein	4 g

Exchanges
1 Starch

Preparation

1. Bring the water to a boil. Add the potatoes, then bring the water to a simmer for 20–25 minutes, or until the potatoes are tender. Remove from heat and drain the water.
2. Add the milk, salt, white pepper, and Roasted Garlic Puree. Use a mixer to combine the ingredients until they are smooth. Serve immediately.

Baked Stuffed Apples

Ingredients

1 cup apple juice
2 oz dried apricot
2 oz dried cranberry
2 oz white raisins
1 Tbsp brown sugar
1 Tbsp honey
4 medium Red Delicious apples

4 Servings
Serving Size: 1 apple half

Calories	262
Calories from Fat	6
Total Fat	1 g
Saturated Fat	0 g
Cholesterol	0 mg
Sodium	7 mg
Carbohydrate	67 g
Dietary Fiber	7 g
Sugars	57 g
Protein	1 g

Exchanges
1/2 Other Carbohydrate
4 Fruit

Preparation

1. Preheat the oven to 300°F. In a small pot, bring the apple juice to a simmer. Add the dried fruit and steep until the fruit is tender, about 3–5 minutes. Remove the fruit and combine with brown sugar and honey.
2. Cut the apples in half and remove the core using a spoon or melon baller. Make sure all the seeds have been removed, but that you leave the bottom and top of the apple intact to keep the fruit from falling out. Spoon the fruit mixture into the centers of the apples. Bake in the oven for 30–35 minutes, or until tender.

Did You Know? A Yale University study discovered that the fragrance of apples will relax a person. In fact, the smell of mulled cider or baked apples actually reduced anxiety attacks. It might be good to bake this dish around the holidays.

$\mathcal{B}$osc Pears Poached in Red Wine

Ingredients

- 4 medium Bosc pears, ripe
- 4 medium oranges, juiced
- 2 Tbsp lemon rind, grated
- 2 Tbsp orange rind, grated
- 1 2/3 cup red wine (such as Cabernet Sauvignon)
- 3 Tbsp honey

---

4 Servings
Serving Size: 1/2 pear

Calories	250
Calories from Fat	10
Total Fat	1 g
Saturated Fat	0 g
Cholesterol	0 mg
Sodium	7 mg
Carbohydrate	46 g
Dietary Fiber	5 g
Sugars	34 g
Protein	2 g

Exchanges
1 Other Carbohydrate
2 Fruit

Preparation

1. Bring water to a boil in a large pot. Add the pears and cook for 15–20 seconds. Remove the pears from the pot and immediately place in a bowl of ice water.
2. Remove the skin from the pears. Slice the pears in half and remove the seeds.
3. Combine the juice of the oranges, the lemon and orange rinds, the red wine, and the honey and bring to a simmer. Add the pears, cover, and cook for 10–20 minutes, or until the pears are tender. Serve each pear with the sauce.

Condiments

Spicy Marinara Sauce

Ingredients

- 2 tsp olive oil
- 1 Tbsp garlic, minced
- 1 cup red bell pepper, thinly sliced
- 1 cup green bell pepper, thinly sliced
- 1 Tbsp jalapeño pepper, minced
- 2 28-oz cans plum tomatoes
- 2 tsp red pepper flakes
- 1/2 cup fresh basil leaves, chopped

10 Servings
Serving Size: about 2/3 cup

Calories	51
Calories from Fat	11
Total Fat	1 g
Saturated Fat	0 g
Cholesterol	0 mg
Sodium	236 mg
Carbohydrate	10 g
Dietary Fiber	2 g
Sugars	5 g
Protein	2 g

Exchanges
2 Vegetable

Preparation

1. Heat the olive oil in a large pot over medium heat. Add the garlic, red and green bell peppers, and jalapeño pepper. Cook until the vegetables are tender, about 5–7 minutes.
2. Drain the liquid from the canned tomatoes into the pot. Crush the plum tomatoes with your hand, then add them to the pot. Stir well to combine, then bring the liquid to a simmer. Add the red pepper flakes and continue to simmer for 20 minutes.
3. Remove the pot from the heat, add the basil leaves, and mix well. Serve or refrigerate for later use.

Red Wine Vinegar with Shallots, Peppercorn, and Rosemary

Ingredients

8 oz red wine vinegar
1/8 cup shallots, peeled
1 tsp black peppercorns
1 sprig fresh rosemary

16 Servings
Serving Size: 1 Tbsp

Calories	.5
Calories from Fat	0
Total Fat	0 g
Saturated Fat	0 g
Cholesterol	0 mg
Sodium	2 mg
Carbohydrate	0 g
Dietary Fiber	0 g
Sugars	0 g
Protein	0 g

Exchanges
none

Preparation

1. Combine all the ingredients into a bottle or jar and seal tightly. Store in the refrigerator.

Flavor Idea: This vinegar imparts a great flavor. Use it sparingly on salads or vegetables, or substitute it for other vinegars in salad dressings.

*T*arragon Butter

Ingredients

1 4-oz stick unsalted butter
2 Tbsp fresh tarragon, chopped
1 tsp lemon rind, grated
1 tsp black pepper, grated

8 Servings
Serving Size: 1 Tbsp

Calories	103
Calories from Fat	103
Total Fat	12 g
Saturated Fat	7 g
Cholesterol	31 mg
Sodium	2 mg
Carbohydrate	0 g
Dietary Fiber	0 g
Sugars	0 g
Protein	0 g

Exchanges
2 Fat

Preparation

1. Allow the butter to soften at room temperature for 30 minutes.
2. Combine the butter with the chopped tarragon, lemon rind, and black pepper.
3. Shape the butter into a small stick and wrap tightly in plastic wrap. This will keep in the refrigerator for up to 2 months.

Basic Pie Pastry

Ingredients

2 1/2 cups all-purpose
       flour
1/4 tsp salt
3 1/2 Tbsp sugar
1/2 cup canola oil
1/4 cup ice water
  2 Tbsp low-fat (1%)
       milk

2 Servings
Serving Size: 1 pie shell

Calories	1143
Calories from Fat	507
Total Fat	56 g
Saturated Fat	4 g
Cholesterol	1 mg
Sodium	303 mg
Carbohydrate	142 g
Dietary Fiber	4 g
Sugars	25 g
Protein	17 g

Exchanges
8 Starch
11 Fat

Preparation

1. Mix the dry ingredients in a bowl. Slowly add the oil and combine with a fork. Slowly add the ice water and milk. Use your hands to form a dough. Separate into two balls, wrap tightly with plastic wrap, and store until needed.

Roasted Tomato Vinaigrette

Ingredients

1/4 lb plum tomatoes
  2 Tbsp balsamic vinegar
  1 Tbsp garlic, minced
1/4 cup extra virgin
     olive oil
1/4 tsp black pepper
1/2 Tbsp fresh oregano,
     chopped

25 Servings
Serving Size: 1 Tbsp

Calories	39
Calories from Fat	36
Total Fat	4 g
Saturated Fat	0 g
Cholesterol	0 mg
Sodium	1 mg
Carbohydrate	1 g
Dietary Fiber	0 g
Sugars	>1 g
Protein	0 g

Exchanges
1 Fat

Preparation

1. Preheat the oven to 350°F. Slice the plum tomatoes in half lengthwise and remove any stem. Bake in the oven for 25–30 minutes, or until the tomatoes are tender and slightly browned. Remove from the oven and allow them to cool.
2. Place the plum tomatoes and balsamic vinegar in a food processor and puree until smooth. Add the garlic and continue to puree. Slowly pour in the olive oil until it is well mixed. Add the black pepper and oregano and mix well.

Flavor Idea: This is not only a great addition to salads, but it makes a nice condiment for fish or meat. Use it sparingly.

Three-Pepper Butter

Ingredients

1 4-oz stick unsalted
   butter
1 tsp black peppercorns
1 tsp red peppercorns
1 tsp Szechwan pepper-
   corns

8 Servings
Serving Size: 1 Tbsp

Calories	103
Calories from Fat	103
Total Fat	12 g
Saturated Fat	7 g
Cholesterol	31 mg
Sodium	2 mg
Carbohydrate	0 g
Dietary Fiber	0 g
Sugars	0 g
Protein	0 g

Exchanges
2 Fat

Preparation

1. Allow the butter to soften at room temperature for 30
   minutes.
2. Heat a small pan over medium heat. Add the peppercorns
   and allow them to toast for 1–2 minutes. Place the peppercorns in a coffee grinder and grind until fine.
3. Combine the butter and the peppercorn mixture and mix
   well. Reshape the butter into a small stick and wrap tightly
   in plastic wrap. This will keep in the refrigerator for
   2 months.

Vanilla Butter

Ingredients

1 4-oz stick unsalted butter
1/2 vanilla bean
1 tsp artificial sweetener
1 tsp cinnamon

8 Servings
Serving Size: 1 Tbsp

Calories	103
Calories from Fat	103
Total Fat	12 g
Saturated Fat	7 g
Cholesterol	31 mg
Sodium	2 mg
Carbohydrate	0 g
Dietary Fiber	0 g
Sugars	0 g
Protein	0 g

Exchanges
2 Fat

Preparation

1. Allow the butter to soften at room temperature for 30 minutes.
2. Slice the vanilla bean lengthwise and scrape the meat from inside the bean.
3. Combine the butter with the vanilla meat, artificial sweetener, and cinnamon. Mix well.
4. Shape the butter into a small stick and wrap tightly in plastic wrap.

Flavor Idea: This butter tastes great not only on the pancakes included earlier (see pp. 34 and 35), but also on toast, waffles, or anything else.

Homemade Chicken Stock

Ingredients

3 lb chicken bones
8 quarts cold water
2 medium onions, diced
1 medium carrot, diced
2 stalks celery, diced
2 bay leaves
1 tsp black peppercorns
1 tsp rosemary
1 tsp thyme

Preparation

1. In a large pot, combine the chicken bones and water and bring to a simmer. Skim and discard any fat that rises to the top of the pot. Simmer for 1 hour.
2. Add the remaining ingredients to the pot. Continue to simmer until the liquid is reduced to 1/4 its original volume, about 3–4 hours. Strain the liquid into a separate bowl and allow it to cool. Refrigerate or freeze for later use.

Chef's Hints: This is the basic recipe that is used widely in this book, but you can always substitute low-sodium chicken broth if you are short on time. Homemade chicken stock is much more flavorful, though, and it contains no calories! Freeze the stock in ice cube trays to make it easier to use later.

Red Onion Confit

Ingredients

2 tsp olive oil
1 lb red onion, sliced
4 Tbsp balsamic vinegar
1 Tbsp orange rind, grated

10 Servings
Serving Size: 1/4 cup

Calories	36
Calories from Fat	1
Total Fat	>1 g
Saturated Fat	0 g
Cholesterol	0 mg
Sodium	2 mg
Carbohydrate	8 g
Dietary Fiber	1 g
Sugars	6 g
Protein	1 g

Exchanges
1 Vegetable

Preparation

1. Heat the olive oil in a large pan over medium heat. Add the red onions. Do not stir. Let the onions turn light brown, then turn and brown on the other side.
2. When the onions are almost done, add the balsamic vinegar and orange rind. Cook for 2–3 minutes, until the liquid is almost gone.

*L*emon Pepper Spice Rub

Ingredients

1 Tbsp red peppercorns
1 Tbsp green peppercorns
1 tsp black peppercorns
1 tsp white peppercorns
2 Tbsp lemon rind, grated

2 Servings
Serving Size: 2 Tbsp

Calories	52
Calories from Fat	18
Total Fat	2 g
Saturated Fat	0 g
Cholesterol	0 mg
Sodium	5 mg
Carbohydrate	11 g
Dietary Fiber	5 g
Sugars	0 g
Protein	2 g

Exchanges
none

Preparation

1. In a coffee grinder, grind the peppercorns until fine. Combine the peppercorns with the lemon zest and mix well. Refrigerate for up to 2 days.

Flavor Idea: This is a great low-fat way to add flavor and spiciness to your meals. Simply rub this spice combination into chicken, meat, or fish, and allow it to sit in the refrigerator for an hour while it absorbs the flavor. Then cook it like you normally would.

$\mathcal{H}$erb Butter

Ingredients

- 1 4-oz stick unsalted butter
- 1/2 tsp fresh thyme, finely chopped
- 1/2 tsp fresh sage, finely chopped
- 1/2 tsp fresh rosemary, finely chopped

8 Servings
Serving Size: 1 Tbsp

Calories	103
Calories from Fat	103
Total Fat	12 g
Saturated Fat	7 g
Cholesterol	31 mg
Sodium	2 mg
Carbohydrate	0 g
Dietary Fiber	0 g
Sugars	0 g
Protein	0 g

Exchanges
2 Fat

Preparation

1. Allow the butter to soften at room temperature for 30 minutes.
2. Combine the butter with the thyme, sage, and rosemary. Mix well.
3. Shape the butter into a small stick and wrap tightly in plastic wrap. This can be stored for up to 3 months.

*E*asy Stuffing

Ingredients

- 2 Tbsp butter
- 1 cup onion, diced
- 1/2 tsp sage
- 1/2 tsp thyme
- 1/2 tsp rosemary
- 1 Tbsp fresh parsley, chopped
- 6 cups dry or day-old bread, cut into 1/2-inch cubes
- 1 1/4 cups Chicken Stock (see p. 155), hot

10 Servings
Serving Size: about 1/2 cup

Calories	84
Calories from Fat	29
Total Fat	3 g
Saturated Fat	2 g
Cholesterol	7 mg
Sodium	238 mg
Carbohydrate	12 g
Dietary Fiber	1 g
Sugars	2 g
Protein	2 g

Exchanges
1 Starch
1/2 Fat

Preparation

1. Preheat the oven to 350°F. Melt the butter in a large pot over medium heat. Add the onions and cook for 3–5 minutes, or until the onions are translucent. Add the sage, thyme, rosemary, and parsley. Cook for 1 minute. Add the bread cubes and half of the chicken stock. Remove the pot from the heat.
2. Gently combine the ingredients. Add the rest of the chicken stock and again mix gently. Place the entire mixture in a baking dish and bake for 30 minutes.

Roasted Garlic Puree

Ingredients

1 garlic bulb
1 tsp olive oil

2 Servings
Serving Size: 2 Tbsp

Calories	60
Calories from Fat	27
Total Fat	3 g
Saturated Fat	>1 g
Cholesterol	0 mg
Sodium	0 mg
Carbohydrate	8 g
Dietary Fiber	0 g
Sugars	0 g
Protein	0 g

Exchanges
1 Fat

Preparation

1. Preheat the oven to 325°F. Slice the top of the garlic bulb so that the garlic pieces are just exposed. Place the bulb on a small baking dish and rub 1 tsp of olive oil over the skin. Put the garlic in the same oven as the beef and bake for 20 minutes, or until the garlic bulb is soft to the touch. Remove the garlic and allow it to cool.
2. Once cool, break open the garlic bulb and squeeze the garlic pulp from the skin. Discard any of the skin or peel. Puree the roasted garlic in a food processor until it is a paste.

Flavor Idea: Not only is this puree a great flavor enhancer for many recipes, but many people enjoy it as a snack. Try a small amount on a cracker or a small piece of toasted bread.

Recipe Index

A

Antipasti Salad, 21

Asparagus Wrapped in Phyllo, 6

B

Baked Catfish Nuggets, 87

Baked Chicken Parmesan, 79

Baked Halibut with Lemon Dill Sauce, 129

Baked Salmon Fish Sticks, 88

Baked Sea Scallops, 15

Baked Spanish Mackerel with Tomato Caper Sauce, 130

Baked Stuffed Apples, 144

Banana and Vanilla Pancakes, 34

Barbecued Chicken Wings, 42

Basic Pie Pastry, 151

Basmati Rice with Lemon and Thyme, 22

Beef Stir-Fry, 5

Black Bean and Orzo Pasta, 124

Blackberry Cobbler, 64

Bosc Pears Poached in Red Wine, 145

Breakfast Hashbrowns, 111

Broiled Lamb Chops with Onion Confit, 86

Buttery String Beans, 142

C

Cajun Baked Sweet Potato, 96

Carrot and Ginger Soup, 18

Chicken and Mushrooms in White Wine Sauce, 7

Chicken Breast Roulade Stuffed with Ham and Goat Cheese, 8

Chicken Cordon Bleu, 77

Chicken Jambo, 9

Chicken Kiev, 116

Chicken Minute Steak Philly, 78

Chicken Pot Pie, 117

Chicken Stir Fry, 80

Chicken Tenders with Roasted Garlic, Mushrooms, and Onions, 44

Chocolate Cake Celebration, 28

Chopped Steak with Pepper Gravy, 73

Corn Salsa, 58

Cornish Game Hen in Herb Butter, 83

Crab Cakes, 50

Subject Index

Orzo Pasta with Baby Shrimp, Sun-Dried Tomatoes, and Sweet Pea Puree, 12
Pan-Seared Flounder Almondine, 53
Poached Salmon with Dill, Cinnamon, and Honeydew Salsa, 89
Salmon Roulade, 14
Sautéed Calamari with Roasted Fennel Cream Sauce and Angel Hair Pasta, 131
Sautéed Lemon Shrimp with Zucchini and Yellow Squash Julienne, 18
Shrimp and Scallop Stew, 90
Shrimp Salad with Dill and Cucumber, 16
Smoked Salmon with Goat Cheese on Baguette Rounds, 17
South Carolina Soft-Shell Crab, 54
Spicy Shrimp with Dijon Sauce and Linguine, 132
Stuffed Flounder over Linguine with Spicy Roasted Red Pepper Puree, 91
Tinfoil-Wrapped Swordfish Steak, 133

Soups
Carrot and Ginger Soup, 19
Cream of Potato Soup, 134
Gazpacho Soup, 55
Grilled Apple Pear Soup, 56
Lentil Soup, 93
Minestrone Soup, 94
Split Pea Soup, 135
Vegetable Soup, 19

Vegetables
Asparagus Wrapped in Phyllo, 6
Buttery String Beans, 142
Cajun Baked Sweet Potato, 96
Corn Salsa, 58
Green Beans with Lemon Pepper, 139
Grilled Herbed Zucchini Halves, 60
Grilled Marinated Potatoes, 61
Grilled Portabello Mushrooms, 59
Lima Bean, Corn, and Green Bean Toss, 23
Orange and Honey Glazed Baby Carrots, 140
Paprika Potatoes, 97
Peas and Pearl Onions, 141
Pizza with Plum Tomato and Basil, 49
Red Onion Confit, 156
Roasted Baby Carrots, 99
Roasted Garlic Mashed Potatoes, 143
Roasted Garlic Puree, 160
Sautéed Julienne Vegetables, 24
Sautéed Spinach, 25

About the American Diabetes Association

The American Diabetes Association is the nation's leading voluntary health organization supporting diabetes research, information, and advocacy. Its mission is to prevent and cure diabetes and to improve the lives of all people affected by diabetes. The American Diabetes Association is the leading publisher of comprehensive diabetes information. Its huge library of practical and authoritative books for people with diabetes covers every aspect of self-care—cooking and nutrition, fitness, weight control, medications, complications, emotional issues, and general self-care.

To order American Diabetes Association books: Call 1-800-232-6733. http://store.diabetes.org (Note: there is no need to use **www** when typing this particular Web address.)

To join the American Diabetes Association: Call 1-800-806-7801. www.diabetes.org/membership

For more information about diabetes or ADA programs and services: Call 1-800-342-2383. E-mail: Customerservice@diabetes.org

To locate an ADA/NCQA Recognized Provider of quality diabetes care in your area: Call 1-703-549-1500 ext. 2202. www.diabetes.org/recognition/Physicians/ListAll.asp

To find an ADA Recognized Education Program in your area: Call 1-888-232-0822. www.diabetes.org/recognition/education.asp

To join the fight to increase funding for diabetes research, end discrimination, and improve insurance coverage: Call 1-800-342-2383. www.diabetes.org/advocacy

To find out how you can get involved with the programs in your community: Call 1-800-342-2383. See below for program Web addresses.

- *American Diabetes Month:* Educational activities aimed at those diagnosed with diabetes—month of November. www.diabetes.org/ADM
- *American Diabetes Alert:* Annual public awareness campaign to find the undiagnosed—held the fourth Tuesday in March. www.diabetes.org/alert
- *The Diabetes Assistance & Resources Program (DAR):* diabetes awareness program targeted to the Latino community. www.diabetes.org/DAR
- *African American Program:* diabetes awareness program targeted to the African American community. www.diabetes.org/africanamerican
- *Awakening the Spirit: Pathways to Diabetes Prevention & Control:* diabetes awareness program targeted to the Native American community. www.diabetes.org/awakening

To find out about an important research project regarding type 2 diabetes: www.diabetes.org/ada/research.asp

To obtain information on making a planned gift or charitable bequest: Call 1-888-700-7029. www.diabetes.org/ada/plan.asp

To make a donation or memorial contribution: Call 1-800-342-2383. www.diabetes.org/ada/cont.asp